We dedicate this book to all of our patients and their families.

Creating Heart Health

Ashish Gupta, M.D. and Vinod Kumar, M.D. F.A.C.C.

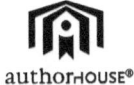

AuthorHouse™
1663 Liberty Drive
Bloomington, IN 47403
www.authorhouse.com
Phone: 1-800-839-8640

© *2011 by Ashish Gupta, M.D. and Vinod Kumar, M.D. F.A.C.C.*
All rights reserved.

No part of this book may be reproduced, stored in a retrieval system, or transmitted by any means without the written permission of the author.

First published by AuthorHouse   10/28/2011

ISBN: 978-1-4678-5868-7 (sc)
ISBN: 978-1-4685-3919-6 (hc)
ISBN: 978-1-4678-5867-0 (ebk)

Printed in the United States of America

Any people depicted in stock imagery provided by Thinkstock are models, and such images are being used for illustrative purposes only.

Certain stock imagery © Thinkstock.

This book is printed on acid-free paper.

Because of the dynamic nature of the Internet, any web addresses or links contained in this book may have changed since publication and may no longer be valid. The views expressed in this work are solely those of the author and do not necessarily reflect the views of the publisher, and the publisher hereby disclaims any responsibility for them.

Table of Contents

Introduction 2-3

Chapter 1: Get to Know Your Heart 5
Heart is just a muscle. And without proper care, muscles break down.

Chapter 2: Heart Disease in the United States 13
After age 40, one out of every two men will develop Coronary Artery Disease.

Chapter 3: Understanding Your Risk 19
Determine your odds of developing a heart attack using the Framingham Risk Analysis.

Chapter 4: From Cholesterol to Homocysteine 27
Learning about your coronary artery disease risk factors.

Chapter 5: The Fabulous Four for Health 35
Prescription for Fabulous Heart Health: healthy diet, get active, quit smoking, and learn to manage stress.

Chapter 6: It's a Family Affair 63
Family history of heart disease puts you at higher risk of developing a heart attack.

Chapter 7: Time for a Test 67
Learning what the most commonly performed tests really mean.

Specific Conditions of the Heart 73

Chapter 8: Atherosclerosis and Heart Attacks 75
By age 40, 70% Americans already have evidence of plaque buildup in their arteries.

Chapter 9: Hypertension 81
70 million Americans suffer from high blood pressure.

Chapter 10: Hyperlipidemia 87
Keep you bad cholesterol (LDL) under 100!

Chapter 11: Diabetes and the Heart 91
Patients with Diabetes are more likely to die of heart disease than from anything else!

Chapter 12: Peripheral Artery Disease 95
Do you have difficulty walking?

Chapter 13: Congestive Heart Failure 99
Is your heart pumping enough blood?

Chapter 14: Atrial Fibrillation 103
Rhythm of your heart matters.

Chapter 15: Graphics 107
Examples of posters and graphics displayed at The Heart Center

Glossary 115

Introduction

You've probably heard a loved one or a doctor tell you numerous times, "John it's time to lose weight" or "Becky, you need to stop smoking, it's killing you!" or "David, stop being a couch potato, it'll make you sick!" But what you probably haven't understood is how important these small advises are to make big differences in not only how long you live, but how well you live.

This book is an effort to give heart patients like yourself, all of the tools you need to make small changes in outlook to drastically improve disease outcome. From 'Getting to Know Your Heart' to understanding the development of the 8 most common cardiac diseases that affect a significant number of Americans today, this book will equip you with all the knowledge you need about your heart and how you can keep it healthy. Easy to follow charts, tables, and pictures will help you extract and apply the vast knowledge contained in the book.

As you go thru this book, you will see how heart attacks are the #1 killers in America. We have included the Framingham Risk Analysis which will help you add up your risk of developing one in the next ten years!

Using simple analogies, we have explained the meaning behind so many of the words we all throw around every day without knowing what they actually mean, like diabetes and hypertension. What will amaze you is that these diseases affect millions of Americans, and you could very well be next, unless you put a foot forward in the right direction.

But what is that right direction?

Well, of course-the Fabulous Four of Health! These are the pillars behind the cardiac reversal program we have developed for our patients. In this program we encourage our patients not only to comply with principles of good evidence based medicine, but add those components which are just as important in predicting disease outcome: diet, physical activity, abstinence from smoking, and managing stress.

We share with you a typical day at the "Good Family, Good Heart" seminar, where you and your spouse are requested to come together and gain from a positive experience of healthy living.

This book will inspire you to act—it will give you simple techniques to put all of this vast knowledge into action. It will motivate you to increase compliance with your medications and practice a healthy lifestyle. Before you know it, you will have made a healthier you, a healthier family, and a healthier Kern County.

So, next time you go out for dinner, take out a few seconds to tell the waiter to be "light on the cheese" because that cheese just might end up going farther than your stomach. It just might be enough to tip the balance and put you in the Emergency Room for a few hours.

We wish you a happy and healthy reading!

Ashish Gupta, M.D.
Vinod Kumar M.D., F.A.C.C.

Get to Know *Your* Heart

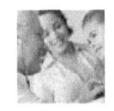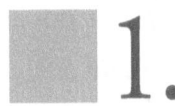

Heart is just a muscle. And without proper care, muscles break down.

With the possible exception of the brain, no other organ in our body carries as much physical and emotional baggage as the heart. In our culture, the heart epitomizes who we are. We call people "soft-hearted" or "hard-hearted," accuse people of "closing their hearts" to others, and say someone died "of a broken heart." We experience "heartache" and "heartbreak" and are "heartfelt" or "heartless." If someone is "hearty," they're full of life and robust. If someone "has heart," they're brave and fearless.

Yet, we treat our heart with such disdain. We smoke, eat fatty meals, don't get enough exercise, and put ourselves in stressful situations — all without the slightest regard for the organ that keeps us going day in and day out. We forget that the heart is, first and foremost, a muscle. And without proper care, muscles break down.

Before we get into all the things that can go wrong with the heart, let's take a minute to examine this most amazing structure, one that will beat an average of 3.3 billion times by the time you're 70.

Your Heart: Just the Basics
How big is my heart?

Close your hand into a fist. There, that's the size of your heart. And yet consider what this small, 10-ounce muscle does 24 hours a day, seven days a week: It pumps — about 1.3 gallons of blood a minute, 1,900 gallons a day, 48 million gallons by the time you hit 70. Try that with your basement sump pump!

The Four Chambers of The Heart
How does my heart pump blood?

The heart is actually two pumps: one on the right, which pumps oxygen-poor blood through the *pulmonary artery* into the lungs to pick up oxygen; and one on the left, which receives that oxygen-rich blood back from the lungs and pumps it out into the rest of the body.

As you can see from the illustration above, the heart is composed of four main chambers through which blood moves:

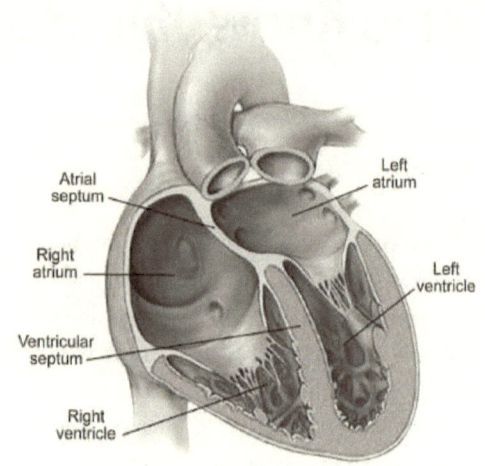

- **Right atrium:**
  Collects oxygen-poor blood from two large veins and contracts to push it into the right ventricle
- **Right ventricle:**
  Contracts to push oxygen-poor blood out of the heart to the lungs
- **Left atrium:**
  Collects oxygen-rich blood from the pulmonary veins and contracts to push it into the left ventricle
- **Left ventricle:**
  Contracts to push oxygen-rich blood out of the heart into the aorta and from there to the rest of the body.

Between each *atrium* and *ventricle* are valves that open and close to let blood in and out. If these valves don't work properly, we run into problems like *mitral valve prolapse*, which you'll learn about later in this book.

I wish I could show you a little movie to demonstrate how blood moves through the heart, but since I can't, you'll have to imagine it from my description.

From the aorta, the larger artery that carries blood from the left ventricle of the heart, the blood passes through your *coronary arteries* to deliver fresh oxygen and other nutrients to the heart itself, then heads out to the rest of your body.

Meanwhile, on the other end, exhausted blood moves back up your body into the heart, drawn there by pressure when the heart contracts, similar to sucking liquid up a straw.

How does my heart beat?

Just as that basement sump pump has to be plugged into an electrical outlet to move the water out of your basement, your heart is also powered by electricity. Instead of plugging into a wall socket, it uses electricity generated by cells that make up its own natural pacemaker, called the sinus, or sinoatrial, node. These cells are called *pacemaker cells*.

They operate like the "wave" at a football game, generating a series of electrical currents that move down the heart, stimulating it to contract in sections, first the upper two chambers, then the lower two chambers, with a slight pause in between. These waves are what we measure during an *electrocardiogram*, or EKG. Ideally, your heart beats according to a steady rhythm, called the sinus rhythm. If there's a glitch in the electrical system, that rhythm gets out of sync. This is called an *arrhythmia*. We'll talk more about arrhythmias later in the book.

The heart normally contracts at about 72 beats a minute. But when you're excited and adrenaline courses through your bloodstream, it signals your sinus node to speed up, increasing the number of beats per minute and sending larger quantities of oxygenated blood through your bloodstream. Conversely, when you're resting, or if you're in really amazing physical shape (think Lance Armstrong) it beats slower. Some medications can have the same effect. Beta blockers, for instance, make your heart beat slower; adrenaline makes it beat faster.

How does blood get to the heart in the first place?

Just one more major part of the heart to discuss: the coronary arteries. These arteries feed blood to the heart. Without oxygenated blood, your heart, like any other tissue in your body, won't work. The arteries have three layers: A smooth, Teflon-like inner layer; a muscular middle layer that contracts with the heart to move blood through; and a tough outer layer, like the casing on a sausage. Although numerous things can go wrong with each layer, it's the interior lining of the artery we're most often concerned with. Here's an analogy I like to use to explain the coronary arteries. Take a rubber band and wrap it around your hand. See how flexible it is? That's how your coronary arteries operate when they're healthy—easily dilating and contracting with no problems. Now take that rubber band and stick it in a glass of ice water and try to stretch and contract it. Notice how stiff it is? What happened to that suppleness? Just as the ice water changed the way the rubber band reacts to stress, so, too, does your lifestyle change the way your coronary arteries behave. What you eat, whether you smoke, and how much you exercise all affect those arteries.

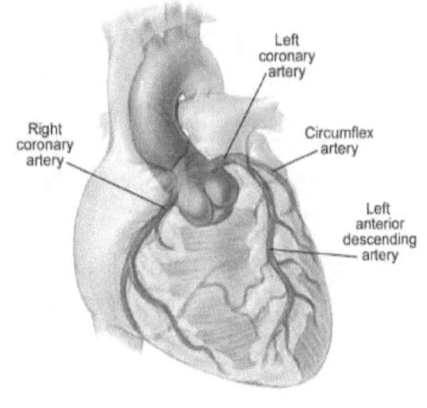

How do my arteries get damaged?

Like any tube that's under a lot of pressure, the artery walls can get damaged. Every time that happens, immune system cells rush in to make repairs. As they try to fix the damage, they create *inflammation*. You know inflammation as the warm, red, throbbing feeling you get after you cut your hand. Inside a coronary artery, inflammation only serves to further damage those artery walls, making them sticky. And, like contractors who don't put down drop cloths when they remodel your bathroom, these immune system cells can create quite a mess, some of which gets carted off, some of which sticks to artery walls.

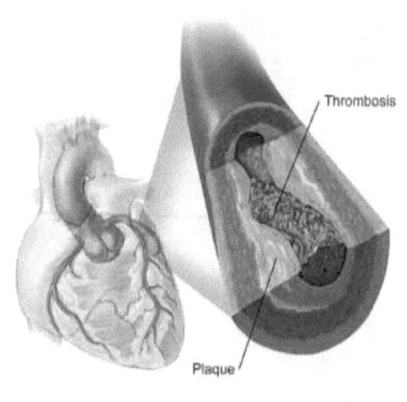

Those sticky artery walls act like flypaper. Instead of capturing insects, they capture cholesterol.

The cholesterol is also sticky, attracting more debris, including cellular junk and calcium. This causes several problems.

First, it narrows the artery, affecting blood flow. As you can imagine, the narrower the artery, the more pressure required to push blood through. This not only increases blood pressure, but increases the risk that the blood flow will knock off a piece of the gunk, or *plaque*, now lining your artery walls. This plaque can block blood flow elsewhere in the artery, causing a *heart attack*. Or, a blood clot could form on top of the plaque, blocking the artery or breaking off and causing a heart attack or stroke.

Once this happens, you're dealing with serious heart disease. Hopefully, by following my recommendations throughout the rest of this book, you can avoid this scenario and maintain a healthy heart for years to come.

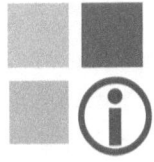

Surprising Facts about the Heart

- Heart muscles contract approximately 100,000 times per day.
- Blood from the heart travels through more than 60,000 miles of vessels before returning to the lungs and heart.
- The heart normally beats 72 times a minute.
- The heart only weighs about 10 ounces.
- By the time you turn 70, your heart will have pumped about 48 million gallons of blood and beaten about 3.3 billion times.

Test Your Knowledge

Answer the following questions to see how much you have learned about your heart. Then turn to the next page for the correct answers.

1. By the time you turn 70, your heart will have beat:
   a. 30 million times
   b. 250 million times
   c. 1.1 billion times
   d. 3.3 billion times

2. Your heart is the size of a:
   a. Cherry
   b. Plum
   c. Fist
   d. Golf ball

3. Your heart pumps 1.3 gallons of blood every:
   a. Second
   b. Minute
   c. Hour
   d. Day

4. The right side of the heart pumps oxygen-poor blood through the pulmonary artery into the:
   a. Lungs
   b. Right side of the heart
   c. Spleen
   d. Rest of the body

5. Match the part of the heart to its correct function:

   1. Right atrium   a. Contracts to push oxygen-poor blood out of the heart to the lungs

   2. Right ventricle   b. Collects oxygen-rich blood from the pulmonary veins and contracts to push it into the left ventricle

   3. Left atrium   c. Collects oxygen-poor blood from two large veins and contracts to push it into the right ventricle

   4. Left ventricle   d. Contracts to push oxygen-rich blood out of the heart into the aorta, and from there to the rest of the body.

6. The heart is powered by:
   a. Blood
   b. Oxygen
   c. Electricity
   d. A pacemaker

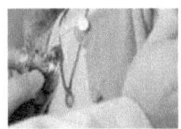

7. A normal, steady heart beat is called the:
   a. Sinus rhythm   b. Arrhythmia
   c. Electrocardiogram d. Sinoatrial node

8. How many layers do arteries have?
   a. 1   b. 2
   c. 3   d. 4

9. Why is plaque dangerous?
   a. It can narrow arteries.
   b. It can break off and block blood flow, causing a heart attack.
   c. It can lead to the formation of a blood clot.
   d. All of the above.

10. A major contributor to heart disease is:
    a. Slow blood flow   b. Inflammation
    c. Electricity   d. Missing arterial layers

Answers:
1. d 2. c 3. b 4. a 5. 1-c, 2-a, 3-b, 4-d 6. c 7. a 8. c 9. d 10. b

Heart Disease in the United States

After age 40, one out of every two men will develop Coronary Artery Disease.

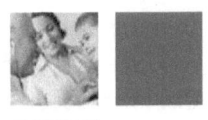

2.

In the last chapter you learned about how your heart works. While this amazing, resilient muscle is designed to last a lifetime, it can and does "get sick." *Cardiovascular disease* refers to conditions affecting the heart and blood vessels; *coronary artery disease* is a type of cardiovascular disease that occurs when the blood vessels that supply blood and oxygen to the heart become narrowed or blocked. Coronary artery disease is also called coronary heart disease, or CHD. While millions of people seek treatment for symptoms of coronary artery disease, it's possible to have the disease and not know it. In fact, between one-fourth and one-half of people who have heart attacks have no symptoms before their attack, a so-called "asymptomatic heart attack." That's why regular medical check-ups are so important!

Cardiovascular heart disease is by far the leading cause of death of both men and women in the United States; even when considered separately from other heart diseases, coronary artery disease is still the leading cause of death in this country. Coronary artery disease is responsible for one out of every five deaths in the United States.

Heart Disease and Women

You probably know that heart disease is the leading cause of death in men, but did you know it's the leading cause of death in women, too? In fact, coronary artery disease is a true "equal opportunity" disease. While women develop coronary artery disease later than men, women are more likely to die of a heart attack than men— 42 percent of women who have a heart attack will die within a year, compared to 24 percent of men. However, it's never too late to reduce your risk of coronary artery disease. Throughout the rest of this book, we'll show you how.

According to the Centers for Disease Control, nearly 16 million people have coronary artery disease and that number is increasing. More than 8.5 million men and 7.2 million women over the age of 20 have been diagnosed with the disease. In 2008, about 700,000 people were expected to have their first heart attack, and another 500,000 would have a recurrent attack. About 20 to 25 percent of all heart attacks are "silent" and do not cause any symptoms.

In those cases, the person doesn't recognize the severity of the condition or doesn't seek treatment for it. In medical terminology, heart attacks are known as myocardial infarctions, or MIs, in which part of the heart muscle is damaged. Although we've gotten much better at treating heart attacks and reducing the risk of dying from one, the best way to make sure you don't die from a heart attack is to prevent it in the first place—which, of course, is what this book is all about.

> **Did You Know?**
>
> If you came into the hospital in the 1950s with a heart attack, you had a 33 percent chance of surviving. Today, your chance of surviving is more than 90 percent.

Coronary Artery Disease and Your Risk

Your total risk of developing coronary artery disease throughout your lifetime is higher if you're a man. After the age of 40, one out of every two men and one out of every three women will develop coronary artery disease. In fact, it's responsible for more than half of all cardiovascular events, including heart attacks, which occur in people under 70.

Your personal risk of developing coronary artery disease, however, depends on several factors. Some are controllable, such as smoking; others aren't, like your family history. Risk factors include the following, most of which I'll cover more in depth later in the book:

- **Age.** The older you are, the more likely you are to develop coronary artery disease. Men who are 45 and older and women who are 55 and older have the greatest risk, and more than 80 percent of those who die from heart disease are 65 or older. Men also tend to develop coronary artery disease earlier and to have heart attacks earlier than women. The average age for a first heart attack in men is 66; in women, it's 70. This all makes sense when you consider that the older you are, the more wear and tear has occurred on your arteries and the longer you've likely been following heart-damaging lifestyle habits. However, heart attacks are becoming more common among people ages 35 to 45. In fact, data from autopsies find that by age 40, up to 70 percent of Americans already have evidence of plaque buildup in their coronary arteries. Why? More people are overweight and sedentary and have increasing daily stresses at home, work, and within relationships.

- **Diabetes.** If you have diabetes, your risk of coronary artery disease is much higher than that of someone without diabetes. That's likely due to the damaging effects of high blood sugar and insulin on coronary arteries.

- **Gender.** For most of your life, just being a man ups your risk of heart disease. Until age 60, men are more likely to have heart attacks than women and are more likely to have heart attacks at a younger age. After age 60, however, women develop coronary artery disease at the same rate as men.
- **Heredity.** If your parents have or had heart disease, you're more likely to develop it than someone whose parents didn't have the disease. The reason? As with any disease, there is some genetic component to heart disease that, coupled with the right environmental factors, increases your risk.
- **High blood pressure.** People with high blood pressure, or *hypertension*, have an increased risk for coronary artery disease. High blood pressure makes the heart work harder, which weakens the muscle over time and can damage blood vessels. The American Heart Association defines high blood pressure in an adult as a blood pressure greater than or equal to 140 mm Hg systolic pressure or greater than or equal to 90 mm Hg diastolic pressure. Ideally, your blood pressure should be no more than 120/80.
- **High cholesterol.** Had your *cholesterol* checked lately? If you have a high blood cholesterol level, called *hypercholesterolemia*, you're more likely to develop coronary artery disease simply because there's more cholesterol in your blood that may stick to artery walls. Here's the thing about cholesterol levels: While your risk of coronary artery disease increases steadily as total blood cholesterol levels exceed 160 mg/dL, doctors use 200 mg/dL as the marker for "borderline high" cholesterol; if it's above 240 mg/dL, it's considered high. That means the lower your cholesterol, the better you are.

One Patient's Story*

Jim was only 35 when he began having chest pains. He went to his regular doctor, who gave him a treadmill test, which measures the activity of the heart under stress. Jim passed that test twice but still felt that something was wrong. Since he had a family history of heart disease, he insisted on seeing a cardiologist and came to me. I suspected Jim had a deeper problem and performed another test called a nuclear heart scan that confirmed my suspicion. An angiogram revealed that all of Jim's coronary arteries were blocked. He underwent immediate quadruple heart bypass surgery to restore blood flow to the heart.

* Patient names have been changed to protect their privacy.

A high amount of low-density lipoprotein (LDL cholesterol) also increases your risk of coronary artery disease. (The level of LDL considered high is 130–159 mg/dL or more, depending on other risk factors.) You'll learn more about cholesterol later in the book. A triglyceride level of 150 mg/dL or higher is also considered high and can contribute to coronary artery disease.

Total Cholesterol Level	Category
Less than 200 mg/dL	Desirable
200–239 mg/dL	Borderline high
240 mg/dL and above	High
LDL Cholesterol Level	**Category**
Less than 100 mg/dL	Optimal
100-129 mg/dL	Near optimal/above optimal
130-159	Borderline high
160-189	High
190 and above	Very high
HDL Cholesterol Level	**Category**
60 and above	High*
Less than 40	Low*

*High HDL is considered protective against CHD. Low HDL is a risk factor for coronary heart disease.
Source: ATP III Guidelines, National, Heart, Lung, and Blood Institute

- **Smoking.** If you smoke, you're much more likely to develop coronary artery disease and to die from it. **Smokers are twice as likely to have a heart attack as nonsmokers** and two to four times more likely than non-smokers to die from that heart attack. Smoking damages blood vessels, increasing the likelihood of fatty buildup on artery walls; makes your blood more likely to clot; and increases blood pressure. Quitting smoking is the easiest way to reduce your risk of heart disease and will have the greatest benefit on your overall health

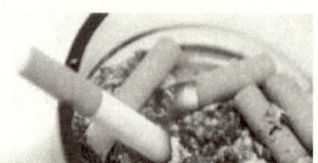

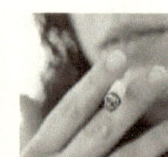

- **Physical activity levels.** Are you a couch potato? Lack of exercise or simple movement increases your risk of heart disease. Exercise helps protect and strengthen your heart as well as helping you maintain a healthy weight, all of which reduce your risk. More on exercise and easy ways to work physical activity into your life later in the book.
- **Weight.** If you're significantly overweight or obese you're more likely to develop coronary artery disease. Excess body fat puts additional strain on the heart. It also contributes to high blood pressure and cholesterol, increases the risk of diabetes, and can keep your body in a highly inflammatory state—all of which increase your risk.
- **Ethnicity.** African Americans are more likely to develop heart disease than whites, while Hispanics are slightly less likely. We don't know exactly why this is; it could be related to certain genetic factors or to lifestyle factors. For instance, African Americans are often under significant chronic stress, a contributing factor to heart disease.

One Patient's Story

Betty, 45, came to me complaining of chest pain. She described it as a "tightening" in her right arm and across her chest and neck. Although she passed a treadmill test, a nuclear heart scan and angiogram revealed that she had a 99 percent blockage in the main artery. I opened the artery with a small balloon, then inserted a stent, a tiny metal scaffolding, in the artery to keep it open. Today she's doing very well.

Test Your Knowledge

Answer the following questions to see how much you have learned about heart disease. Then turn to the next page for the correct answers.

1. **The leading cause of death in women is:**
   a. Breast cancer
   b. Heart disease
   c. Lung cancer
   d. High blood pressure

2. **A heart attack in which part of the heart is damaged is called a(n):**
   a. Myocardial infarction
   b. Arrhythmia
   c. Stroke
   d. Angioplasty

3. **In the United States, more women die of heart attacks than men.**
   a. True
   b. False

4. **All of the following are risk factors for heart disease except:**
   a. Smoking
   b. Family history
   c. Arthritis
   d. Obesity

Answers: 1. b, 2. a, 3. a, 4. c

Understanding Your Risk

Determine your odds of developing a heart attack using the Framingham Risk Analysis.

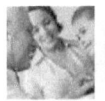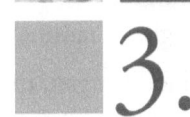

So, now you know about heart disease and its associated risk factors. But just how large a factor do these conditions play? In other words, how do you "add up" your risk factors to determine your personal risk for heart disease?

In this chapter, I'll show you how to determine your own odds of a *heart attack* using a rating system called the **Framingham Risk Analysis**. The results will provide a personalized guideline regarding your potential risk for heart disease. Based on the result, we can develop a strategic, specialized plan to help lower your risk for heart disease or maintain your already low risk for developing the condition.

Heart Attacks

Every year, an estimated 1.2 million people in the United States have a heart attack. Nearly 40 percent die (460,000). Of those fatal attacks, half die within an hour after the first symptom. A heart attack occurs when *plaque* lining the arteries bursts open. Blood cells called platelets rush in to repair the spot where the plaque ruptured, creating blood clots that can block blood flow.

If the area of the heart around the blocked artery doesn't receive enough oxygen-enriched blood, it dies. This is known as a heart attack or *myocardial infarction* (MI). The word *myocardial* means "heart muscle," and *infarction* means "tissue death due to lack of oxygen."

Until fairly recently, we knew little about how and why heart disease developed. Then came the Framingham Heart Study. The National Health Institute, now the National Heart, Lung, and Blood Institute (NHLBI), part of the National Institutes of Health (NIH), instituted the study in 1948. The goal was to identify the most common factors for heart disease by tracking thousands of healthy people over time.

The study's first group of 5,209 participants between ages 30 and 62 were recruited in Framingham, Massachusetts (hence the name, Framingham Heart Study).

Researchers evaluated the participants' physical health and lifestyles—everything from diet to exercise to stress levels—to identify symptoms and risk factors common to heart disease. Participants updated their information every two years.

In 1971, the study was updated in conjunction with Boston University, and a second group of participants joined, made up of children and their spouses from the first group. In 2001, a third group entered—the grandchildren of the original Framingham participants.

Since it began, the Framingham Heart Study has identified numerous heart disease risk factors, including high blood pressure, high *cholesterol*, obesity, physical inactivity, smoking, and diabetes. The study also helped correlate the effect of related risk factors such as triglyceride and cholesterol levels, age, and gender.

These findings remained strong regardless of race and ethnicity, leading to what we know today about heart disease. The study also produced the Framingham Risk Analysis, which I and other doctors commonly use with our patients to assess their risk of heart disease.

The Framingham Risk Analysis

The Framingham Risk Analysis determines your short-term (10-year) risk for heart disease based on your age, cholesterol levels, blood pressure, diabetes status, and smoking status. The results provide a risk prediction based on the risk of the Framingham participants who match your profile. In other words, people like you.

Originally, the equation only predicted the risk of having a heart attack in the next 10 years. However, in 1991, the equation was updated to include the risk of *all coronary artery disease* conditions, including *angina*, in the next decade. Angina is recurring chest pain due to a lack of blood supply to the heart. It results from blocked arteries and often predicts a heart attack. The Framingham equation was also updated to differentiate risks for men and women.

Keep in mind that the Framingham Risk Analysis only applies to people without known heart disease, and it only predicts the likelihood of developing coronary heart disease, not other cardiovascular conditions like heart failure. While this quiz will certainly help you assess your risk, the analysis shouldn't be used in place of any medical checkup or consultation with Dr. Kumar or other doctors!

Using the Framingham Risk Analysis

It's easy to use the Framingham Risk Analysis. You answer questions regarding your lifestyle, age, and blood cholesterol numbers (both *high-density lipoproteins* [HDL] and *low-density lipoproteins* [LDL]). Each answer is then assigned a score, and you add the scores to determine your overall rating.

With that rating, you can compare your risk to a similar man or woman from the Framingham study.

If you currently *do not* have heart disease, answer the following questions to learn your Framingham risk factor.

1. How old are you?

Age (in years)	Points for women
30–34	-9
35–39	-4
40–44	0
45–49	3
50–54	6
55–59	7
60–64	8
65–69	8
70–74	8

2. What is your LDL cholesterol?

(mg/dL)	(mmol/L)	Points for men	Points for women
<100	<2.59	-3	-2
100–129	2.60-3.36	0	0
130-159	3.37-4.14	0	0
160-189	4.15-4.91	1	2
>190	>4.92	2	2

3. What is your HDL cholesterol?

(mg/dL)	(mmol/L)	Points for men	Points for women
<35	<0.90	2	5
35-44	0.91-1.16	1	2
45-49	1.17-1.29	0	1
50-59	1.30-1.55	0	0
.60	.1.56	-1	-2

4. **What is your blood pressure?** (Find the point at which your higher [*systolic*] and lower [*diastolic*] numbers meet).

Systolic (mm Hg)	Diastolic (M / W)	(mm Hg)	Points for men | women
	<80	80–84	
<120	0 / -3		
120-129		0 / 0	
130-139			1 / 0
140-149			2 / 2
>160			3 / 3

5. **Do you have diabetes?**
   Yes — 2 points for men; 4 points for women
   No — 0 points

6. **Do you smoke?**
   Yes — 2 points for men; 2 points for women
   No — 0 points

Add up your point total for questions 1 through 6. Then use your total points to determine your risk according to the chart below. The percentage refers to your risk of developing heart disease in the next 10 years.

One Patient's Story

Brent, 58, came to The Heart Center in 1999 with symptoms of indigestion and gas. His stress test was normal. He had a nuclear scan, which led to an angiogram, which showed a nearly completely blocked main artery. I performed angioplasty and inserted a stent. Within a few days, all of Brent's symptoms were gone, and he was back at work and in good health. "I was very pleased to see how concerned and attentive Dr. Kumar was," Brent says. "There are not too many doctors that take the time and effort to listen."

Men

Point total	10-year risk
Less than or equal to -3	1%
-2	2%
-1	2%
0	3%
1	4%
2	4%
3	6%
4	7%
5	9%
6	11%
7	14%
8	18%
9	22%
10	27%
11	33%
12	40%
13	47%
More than or equal to 14	More than or equal to 56%

Women

Point total	10-year risk
Less than or equal to -2	1%
-1	2%
0	2%
1	2%
2	3%
3	3%
4	4%
5	5%
6	6%
7	7%
8	8%
9	9%
10	11%
11	13%
12	15%
13	17%
14	20%
15	24%
16	27%
More than or equal to 17	More than or equal to 32%

If you like, you can compare yourself to an "average" man or woman. Find your own results in appropriate chart by gender, and find how you rate compared to the rest of the nation.

The "average" man

Age (in years)	Average 10-year risk	Low 10-year risk
30–34	3%	2%
35-39	5%	3%
40-44	7%	4%
45-49	11%	4%
50-54	11%	4%
55-59	16%	7%
60-64	21%	9%
65-69	25%	11%
70-74	30%	14%

The "average" woman

Age (in years)	Average 10-year risk	Low 10-year risk
30–34	Less than 1%	Less than 1%
35-39	1%	Less than 1%
40-44	2%	2%
45-49	5%	3%
50-54	8%	5%
55-59	12%	7%
60-64	12%	8%
65-69	13%	8%
70-74	14%	8%

How did you do? If your risk is low, that's great. If it's higher than you'd like, keep in mind that we can work together both medically and through lifestyle changes to reduce your risk. And remember that calculating your Framingham risk factor is only one step in taking better care of your health and is no substitute for maintaining healthy habits and come in for a check up when necessary.

Test Your Knowledge

Answer the following questions to see how much you learned about the Framingham Risk Analysis. Then turn to the next page for the correct answers.

1. **A heart attack occurs when:**
    a. Plaque clogs a blood vessel
    b. A blood clot clogs a blood vessel
    c. Blood cannot get to the heart
    d. All of the above

2. **The Framingham Risk Analysis is named for:**
    a. The first participant in the trial
    b. The town where the study began
    c. The researcher who conducted the trial
    d. The disease it was designed to study

3. **The Framingham Risk Analysis evaluates all of the following except:**
    a. Weight
    b. Cholesterol level
    c. Age
    d. Blood pressure

4. **Angina is:**
    a. A blocked artery
    b. A mild heart attack
    c. Chest pain due to a lack of blood supply
    d. Dizziness

5. **You can take the Framingham Risk Analysis even if you already have heart disease.**
    a. True   b. False

Answers:
1. d; 2. b; 3. a; 4. c; 5. b

From Cholesterol to Homocysteine:
Learning about Your Coronary Artery Disease Risk Factors

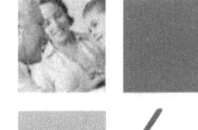

So far, you've learned how common heart disease is in the United States and, if you took the Framingham Risk Analysis, your own risk of having a heart attack in the next 10 years. As you now know, certain risk factors such as age, race, family history, and gender can't be changed. But other risk factors, such as smoking, obesity, and physical inactivity can be altered through lifestyle changes. Changing these parts of your life alters certain markers for heart disease, like high blood pressure, high cholesterol, diabetes, and inflammation. Even if you've already been diagnosed with heart disease, measuring and tracking these risk factors can significantly reduce your risk of having a heart attack or dying of the disease. That's why regular checkups and talking to your doctors about your health are so important. In this chapter, we take a close look at some of the contributing factors to coronary heart disease and heart attacks.

Calcium Plaque

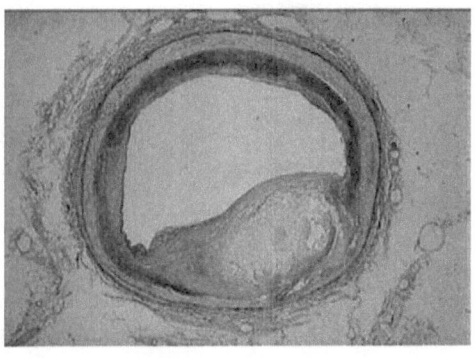

What is it? Calcium is a substance that, together with fat, cholesterol, and dead cells, makes up plaque. As *plaque* thickens and hardens on artery walls, it causes *atherosclerosis*, or a buildup of plaque on artery walls. You may have heard this called "hardening of the arteries" because the more plaque lining the walls, the less flexible the arteries. This can increase blood pressure, as well as limit blood flow through your arteries.

What should I know? A buildup of plaque in your arteries increases your risk of a heart attack and of dying from heart disease.

What can I do? Your doctor can detect coronary calcium with a test called a *computed tomography scan, or CT scan.* It uses X-rays to create a cross-sectional picture of your heart. Depending on the degree of calcium plaque buildup, further tests may be performed to evaluate the narrowing of the *coronary arteries.*

Cholesterol

What is it? Cholesterol is a fatty substance found in animal products and in some vegetable oils such as coconut oil. It's also found in people's blood, where it comes from two primary sources—your liver and your diet.

LDL = "Bad" cholesterol ("L" stands for Lousy)
HDL = "Good" cholesterol ("H" stands for Happy)

There are two primary types of cholesterol: LDL (low-density lipoprotein) and HDL (high-density lipoprotein). Low-density lipoprotein cholesterol is called the "bad" cholesterol (think of the "L" as standing for "lousy") because high levels are associated with an increased risk of heart disease. This form of cholesterol gets deposited on and within the walls of your arteries, contributing to plaque. High-density lipoprotein cholesterol is considered the "good" cholesterol (think of the "H" as standing for "happy") because it helps transport LDL cholesterol back to the liver, where it's broken down and excreted when you go to the bathroom. It may also help remove excess cholesterol from artery walls. As a result, high levels of LDL cholesterol and low levels of HDL cholesterol (high LDL/HDL ratio) are risk factors for atherosclerosis. Conversely, low levels of LDL cholesterol and high levels of HDL cholesterol (low LDL/HDL ratio) reduce your risk of heart disease.

Total Cholesterol Level	Category
Less than 200 mg/dL	Desirable
200–239 mg/dL	Borderline high
240 and above	High

A high LDL on its own also increases your risk of heart disease.

LDL Cholesterol Level	LDL Cholesterol Category
Less than 100 mg/dL	Optimal
100–129 mg/dL	Near optimal/above optimal
130–159 mg/dL	Borderline high
160–189 mg/dL	High
190 mg/dL and above	Very high

What should I know? Your risk of heart disease increases steadily as total blood cholesterol levels exceed 160 mg/dL. That means the lower your cholesterol, the better; but doctors don't classify total blood cholesterol as "borderline high" until it's passed the 200 mg/ dL mark. It's considered "high" when it's above 240 mg/dL. With HDL cholesterol, however, higher numbers are a good thing—an HDL level of 60 mg/dL or higher reduces your risk of heart disease. So reducing your LDL cholesterol and increasing your HDL cholesterol through diet, exercise, and medication can minimize the amount of plaque on artery walls, widen narrowed arteries, and reduce your risk of a heart attack.

What can I do? If you have high cholesterol, losing weight and following a diet low in *saturated fat* can help reduce cholesterol levels. Regular exercise also helps lower LDL cholesterol and increase HDL levels. There are also medicines to bring your cholesterol levels into a better balance. The most commonly used are statins. You'll learn more about statins later in the book.

Diabetes

What is it? Diabetes is a condition in which your body either doesn't make enough insulin or doesn't respond to insulin the way it should. Insulin is a hormone that acts like a doorman at a hotel. Only instead of allowing guests through the lobby doors, it allows glucose, or blood sugar, through a cell's membranes so it can be used to make energy. Without sufficient insulin, your cells don't get the glucose they need and you feel weak and tired. The glucose remains in your blood, damaging blood vessels and various organs. This is where the term "high blood sugar" comes from.

There are two major forms of diabetes—type 1 and type 2. With type 1, your body's insulin-making cells in the pancreas no longer work. People with type 1 diabetes must inject themselves with insulin to survive. This type of diabetes is an *autoimmune* disease that typically strikes in childhood or adolescence.

Type 2 diabetes is much more common, typically occurring in people over 30. With this form of diabetes, your body still produces insulin, but your cells can't use it properly. In many cases, diet and exercise are enough to reverse the disease. Often, however, you need oral medications or injectable insulin. If you don't closely monitor your diabetes and maintain blood sugar levels as close to normal as possible, you significantly increase your risk of heart disease.

What should I know? Anyone can develop diabetes, but you're more likely to get it if your parents have it. Your risk also increases if you're overweight or obese or of American-Indian, Alaskan-Native, African-American or Hispanic descent.

Millions of people have a condition called pre diabetes, in which their blood sugar levels are higher than normal but not high enough to be diagnosed as diabetes. Without significant lifestyle changes, most people with pre diabetes will develop type 2 diabetes within 10 years.

Diabetes can lead to numerous complications, including kidney disease, nerve damage, and blindness. If you have diabetes, you're also at higher risk of developing heart disease or stroke because high blood sugar levels can damage your heart and blood vessels. In addition, people with diabetes are more likely to be overweight or obese, to have high cholesterol, and to have high blood pressure, all of which increase the risk of heart disease. However, up to half of people with diabetes have no symptoms of blocked arteries.

What can I do? Type 2 diabetes often has no symptoms in its early stages, so regular blood glucose screenings are important if you have risk factors. See your doctor immediately if you experience symptoms such as major thirst, frequent urination, weight loss, and blurry eyesight.

Changing your diet, losing weight, and becoming more physically active can all help reduce blood sugar levels and make your cells more responsive to insulin. If you're diagnosed with pre diabetes or diabetes, talk to your doctor about how you can maintain normal blood sugar levels.

One Patient's Story

Jay was 33 and had diabetes for four years. He underwent a stress test after he complained of indigestion. His stress test was normal, but because of his continued symptoms, he underwent a nuclear scan at The Heart Center. That led to an angiogram, which showed significant blockage in his heart arteries. Jay required quadruple coronary bypass surgery. This surgery bypasses the blocked area in the arteries using a new vein or an existing artery so that oxygen-rich blood continues to flow beyond the blocked area to the heart muscles. Jay now is doing well and living a normal life.

High blood pressure

What is it? *Hypertension*, or high blood pressure, occurs when the pressure of the blood inside your large arteries is too high. It is recorded as two numbers. The top number is your *systolic pressure*, which measures the heartbeat that pushes blood out; the bottom number is the *diastolic pressure*, measuring the pressure when your heart relaxes between beats, allowing blood in. Normal blood pressure is 120/80 mm Hg (millimeters of mercury) or less. Hypertension is diagnosed if your blood pressure is consistently above 140 systolic or 90 diastolic (140/90), or both. Blood pressure between 120/80 and 140/90 is considered "prehypertension." The higher your blood pressure—and the longer you have it—the greater your risk of heart disease.

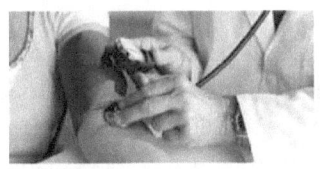

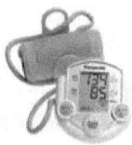

What should I know? Hypertension is very common, affecting 70 million people in the United States. You're more likely to develop high blood pressure as you age and/or if you're African American. High blood pressure is often called a "silent" killer because there are no symptoms. The only way to diagnose it is with regular blood pressure measurements.

We don't know exactly what causes high blood pressure, but there is likely some genetic component. If your parents had it, you're more likely to have it. Your lifestyle also affects your risk. Smoking, drinking excessive amounts of alcohol, and inactivity all tend to increase blood pressure, as does being overweight. However, following a diet high in fruits and vegetables and low in saturated fats and salt, getting regular exercise, not smoking, maintaining a healthy weight, and limiting alcohol intake can all reduce your risk.

What can I do? First, make sure to have your blood pressure checked regularly. You should sit quietly for several minutes before it's measured. Don't have it done if you're angry, upset, or nervous, as that can cause a temporary spike. If your blood pressure is high, talk to your doctor about lifestyle changes (like diet, exercise, and relaxation techniques) and medications to bring it down to normal levels.

Homocysteine

What is it? *Homocysteine* is an amino acid that is normally present in your body. Higher than normal levels (5–15 µmol/L) in your blood are linked to an increased risk of heart disease. This is because homocysteine is a marker for inflammation, which, as you learned, is how your body responds to injury or infection. If homocysteine levels are high, it means there's a lot of inflammation going on somewhere in your body. This type of chronic systemic inflammation increases your risk of developing arterial plaque, in turn raising risk of heart disease.

What should I know? Although we know that high homocysteine levels are a risk factor for heart disease, we don't know for sure that reducing homocysteine levels lowers your risk of a heart attack.

What should I do? Ask your doctor to check your homocysteine blood level. If it's high, your doctor may suggest changing your diet or taking folic acid or other B vitamin supplements. A diet high in foods like leafy green vegetables, fruits, legumes, and whole grains may also help reduce homocysteine levels.

Triglycerides

What are they? *Triglycerides* are blood fats that appear shortly after eating; eventually they're converted into cholesterol. Even a single high fat, high calorie meal can send your triglyceride levels skyrocketing! Triglycerides are one of the four parameters checked when you have a "cholesterol" test: total cholesterol, LDL cholesterol, HDL cholesterol, and triglycerides. Because triglycerides make up the greatest percentage of fat in your blood, people with high triglyceride levels tend to have high overall cholesterol levels, as well.

What should I know? While doctors put more emphasis on total and LDL cholesterol levels, high triglyceride levels (150 mg/dL or higher) also appear to increase your risk of developing heart disease.

What can I do? Lifestyle changes such as losing weight; eating more fruits, vegetables, and whole grains, and fewer saturated fats; and getting regular exercise can all help reduce triglyceride levels. The steps you take to lower your total cholesterol also help lower your triglycerides.

Stay tuned! We'll be covering all those steps in future chapters.

Test Your Knowledge

Answer the following questions to see how much you learned about the various risk factors for heart disease. Then turn to the next page for the correct answers.

1. **A good test for detecting coronary calcium is:**
    a. A stress test
    b. A CT scan
    c. A blood test
    d. An MRI

2. **LDL cholesterol:**
    a. Is considered the "good" cholesterol
    b. Can stick to artery walls
    c. Typically falls as you gain weight
    d. Increases blood pressure

3. **HDL cholesterol:**
    a. Is considered the "good" cholesterol
    b. Can stick to artery walls
    c. Appears in your blood soon after eating
    d. Increases blood pressure

4. **The ideal total blood cholesterol is less than:**
    a. 200 mg/dL
    b. 220 mg/dL
    c. 240 mg/dL
    d. 260 mg/dL or higher

5. **What is a desirable level of LDL cholesterol?**
    a. 100 mg/dL
    b. 131 mg/dL
    c. 148 mg/dL
    d. 170 mg/dL

6. **An ideal HDL cholesterol level is:**
    a. 30 or higher
    b. 40 or higher
    c. 50 or higher
    d. 60 or higher

7. **The best way to diagnose type 2 diabetes is with a(n)**
    a. Blood test
    b. X-ray
    c. Physical examination
    d. Urine test

Continue on next page

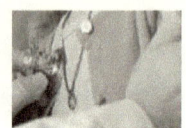

8. The systolic pressure measures:
    a. The pressure that pushes blood out from the heart
    b. The pressure when your heart relaxes between beats
    c. Your risk of heart disease
    d. Your calcium plaque level

9. Homocysteine levels measure which heart disease risk factor?
    a. High blood pressure
    b. Inflammation
    c. Calcium plaque
    d. High cholesterol

10. Triglycerides are blood fats that appear soon after eating.
    a. True   b. False

Answers:
1. b 2. b 3. a 4. a 5. a 6. d 7. a 8. a 9. b 10. a

The Fabulous Four for Health

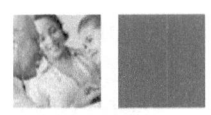

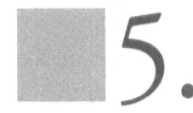

Prescription for Fabulous Heart Health: Healthy diet, Get active, Quit smoking, and Manage stress.

Although you can't change certain risk factors for *cardiovascular disease*, such as your age, gender, and family history, you can reduce your overall risk with lifestyle changes. In this chapter, you'll learn how modifying your diet, becoming physically active, quitting smoking, and managing stress can improve your overall health and reduce your risk of developing heart disease. Even if you've already been diagnosed with some form of heart disease, these changes can help prevent the disease from getting worse and enable you to maintain a better quality of health in years to come.

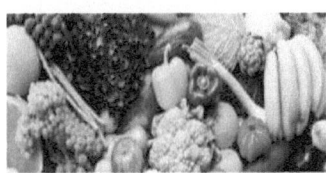

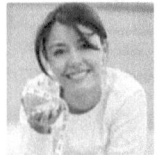

Eat Healthy for Your Heart

You may have heard the common phrases: "You are what you eat," and "You live to eat or eat to live." Eating is an important part of our lives. Our bodies need food and energy to grow and function.

Today, we know more about nutrition than ever before. Yet, despite this knowledge, 68 percent of U.S. adults and 30 to 40 percent of children are overweight or obese, and the numbers continue to rise.

Why is that a problem? The American Heart Association (www.heart.org) says that if you are obese, you are at higher risk for health problems, including high blood pressure, high blood cholesterol and triglycerides, diabetes, heart disease, and stroke.

Obesity by itself is also a proven independent risk factor for heart disease. And not only does obesity adversely affect our heart and blood vessels, it affects almost every other organ of the body.

Studies have shown a connection between obesity and the following health problems:
- Early death
- Heart attack, stroke, or other cardiovascular disease
- Diabetes
- Cancer of the colon, kidney, breast, endometrium, or stomach
- Osteoarthritis
- Dementia
- Insulin resistance
- Hepatobiliary disease
- Urinary incontinence
- Psychosocial dysfunction
- Gastroesophageal reflux disease (GERD)
- Gallstones
- Infertility
- Adult asthma
- Snoring
- Sleep apnea
- Cataracts
- Poorer quality of life

The list goes on…

On the flip side, eating a nutritious diet and maintaining a healthy weight has many benefits, including:
- Longer life
- Significantly lower risk for many chronic diseases including cardiovascular disease, some cancers, diabetes, GERD, asthma, and arthritis
- Stronger immune system
- Better quality of life
- Less disability
- Feeling better
- Looking better
- More energy

The food you eat changes from macro nutrients to micro nutrients as it is digested. Then it crosses the intestinal wall and goes into your blood. The blood carries the nutrients as a sort of a nutrient broth to your cells. These cells use the vital nutrients for metabolism creating energy, life, and thus new cells. It is important to eat right so that your cells get the right nutrients.

> **Putting Fuel in Your Tank**
> Would you put low-octane gas into a high-performance car? Then why would you put less than high-octane fuel into your high-performance body?

So what exactly are these nutrients that we need?

- **1. Macronutrients**
  Carbohydrates
  Proteins
  Fats

- **2. Micronutrients**
  Vitamins*
  Minerals*
  Amino Acids
  Essential Fatty Acids

- **3. Others**
  Fiber*
  Water*

Calories in foods are as follows:	
Carbohydrates	4kcal/gm
Proteins	4kcal/gm
Fats	9kcal/gm

* Other nutrients like fiber, water, vitamins and minerals have no calories.

What to Eat

Our knowledge of what to eat evolved over thousands of years based upon the availability of foods and our ability to produce food. From hunter gatherer, man settled and started agriculture several thousand years ago. However over the last 200 years, our eating habits changed very fast due to industrialization, population shifts into cities and ours ability to preserve foods. Speed of change became even faster over the last century due to progressive shifts in life style and factors of globalization.

In the 1940s, dietary guidelines from the U.S. Department of Agriculture (USDA) promoted eating from each of the seven major food groups. Butter and fortified margarine counted as one of the daily food groups. In addition, the guidelines said, "Eat any other foods you want."

From the mid-1950 into the 1980s, the USDA promoted the Basic 4 concept, which called for **four major food groups** and eating a minimum amount from each of the groups. These guidelines placed less emphasis on meats and saturated fats, but still encouraged Americans to eat several portions of meat a day.

In 1992, the USDA released its classic food pyramid, which attempted to illustrate how much food should come from the various food groups. Grains (bread, cereal, rice, and pasta) anchored the base of the pyramid. Fruits and vegetables came next, followed by smaller portions of dairy and meat, poultry, fish, beans, eggs, and nuts. Fats, oils, and sweets topped the pyramid with the caution to "use sparingly." The pyramid included a suggested serving size for each food group. In 2005, the pyramid underwent a visual makeover, using colorful vertical wedges to represent the portion of each food group. Exercise also entered the picture with an image of a person climbing stairs and a subtitle that said "Steps to a Healthier You."

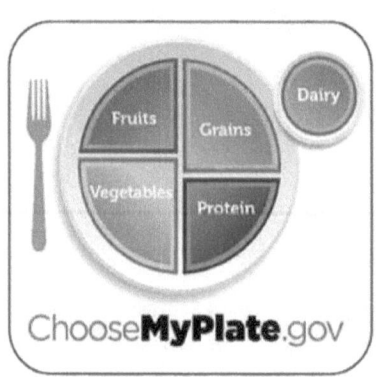

Finally, in 2010, the USDA released **MyPlate**, a simple visual representation of a healthy plate. MyPlate clearly shows that half of your plate should be filled with fruits and vegetables, about one-fourth with grains and one-fourth with proteins, accompanied by a serving of dairy.

We at The Heart Center, Bakersfield, CA have developed a food pyramid for heart patients in which vegetables occupy the largest share of the diet, followed by fruits and then whole grains. Poultry and meat are atop the pyramid, along with approximate caloric values for each to make it much easier to quickly calculate the total calories eaten.

Looking back at these guidelines of the last 70 years, we can see that there has been a gradual shift away from high-calorie, high fats animal-based protein, towards a plant-based nutrition. Research has shown that plant-based diets reduce our risk of common diseases like obesity, heart disease, cancer, and many others. Most of these changes align us with a path that takes us closer to nature, closer to what is natural.

Dr. T. Colin Campbell, a nutrition and health researcher, conducted a 20-year study on diets in rural China. In his book, The China Study, he writes:

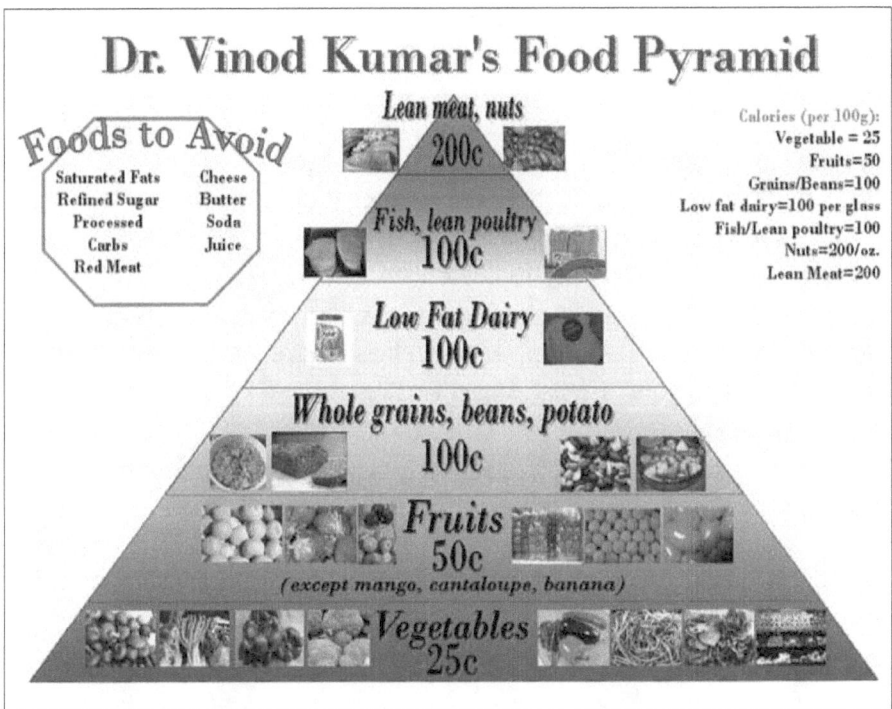

"People who ate the most animal-based foods got the most chronic disease. Even relatively small intakes of animal-based food were associated with adverse effects. People who ate the most plant-based foods were the healthiest and tended to avoid chronic disease." Numerous other researchers have come to similar conclusions.

One of the best-known is Dr. Dean Ornish, founder and president of the Preventive Medicine Research Institute and author of six best-selling books, including Dr. Dean Ornish's Program for Reversing Heart Disease.

Three Simple Steps to help you Eat Right:

1. **Cut Out The Junk Food.**

Eliminate soft drinks, chips, fast food, pastries, cakes, and candy. These foods are high calorie and low nutrition. They are what we call "empty calories". It's OK to have an occasional treat, but balance it out the next day by eating healthier foods. Reduce your intake of foods containing added salts, sugars, and fats. You do not need to add these substances from the outside.

Natural, whole foods have ample amounts of salts, sugars, and fats and are sufficient for body needs. Processed and refined foods tend to have these substances in large quantities, along with other unhealthy additives.

How much salt is good for you?

Sodium, the essential mineral in salt is necessary to transmit nerve impulses and helps to maintain fluid balance in the body. A normal whole foods diet contains about 500 milligrams of salt. RDA recommends up to 1500 mg per day, about ½ teaspoonful of salt and a maximum of 2400 mg of sodium or 6 grams of salt or one teaspoon per day.

The problem is that the modern diet simply has too much salt or sodium and excessive amounts of sodium can contribute to hypertension (high blood pressure). The average American diet consumes about 3,500 milligrams of sodium or 10 grams of salt per day. This comes mainly from the added salt and from processed foods. Many foods contain salt that you may not be aware of such as sauces, dressings, and even soft drinks.

The best you can do is moderation in salt intake, avoid processed foods and avoid added salt as much as possible. Also eat a variety of high- potassium plant foods such as fruits and vegetables.

2. **Eat Whole Foods.**

Whole foods refer to foods in their natural state—not processed, canned, or preserved. Try to eat more fresh or frozen vegetables and fruit, whole grains, and fat-free or low-fat milk and other dairy products.

3. **Improve the quality of your foods.**

Quality of food is too often overlooked. However, quality is essential. As your body uses the macronutrients and micronutrients from the food you eat, it also takes in the pesticides, growth hormones, artificial flavorings, dyes, and other additives including excess salts, sugars and fats. They then make their way to your cells.

Here are some simple guidelines for improving the quality of your food:

- **Eat natural.** This means eat more plant-based foods in the raw state. Processing removes many of the nutrients, vitamins, and antioxidants and may add a lot of unnecessary calories in the form of fats and sugars.
- **Eat fresh.** Each day that food is not eaten it loses valuable vitamins, minerals, and phytochemicals. Food is often picked from the farm five days before it is sold and then sits at home in your refrigerator for some more time after that.
- **Eat local.** Food that is locally grown will need minimum transportation, will be fresher and will likely have fewer additives, which are usually added to preserve freshness and taste. If you eat in accord with what nature produces, you may help your body and the environment.
- **Eat organic.** A century ago almost all food was grown organically. Today organic food is harder to find and often more expensive, but you should strive to eat foods without pesticides, additives, or chemicals. Food Inc., is a great documentary about how our seeds are being genetically modified so that the total amount of food produced is more per acre. If you can't go totally organic, focus on areas where there is a greater chance of pesticide contamination. Try to find the following foods grown organically: nectarines, celery, pears, peaches, apples, cherries, strawberries, imported grapes, spinach, potatoes, bell peppers, and raspberries.
- **Eat colors.** Choose a variety of different colored fruits and vegetables. The various color pigments in the foods boost your immunity, have antioxidant properties and contain vital vitamins and minerals. For example, red foods like tomatoes and watermelon contain lycopene, a carotenoid that may reduce your risk of heart disease, diabetes and some types of cancer. Spinach, which gets its green color from chlorophyll, is rich in health-boosting antioxidants, as well as calcium and iron.
- **Eat at home.** You can more easily control the quality of your food when you eat at home. With wise shopping and healthy cooking techniques, you can ensure you are eating a heart-healthy diet. Try to limit eating out. Check the menu if it includes boiled, steamed, baked or grilled entrées.
- **Minimize meats and fats.** If you eat meat, limit foods high in saturated fats and cholesterol. Look for lean cuts of red meats, pork, and poultry and watch your portion sizes. You can eat moderate amounts of eggs and seafood. Consume small quantities of monounsaturated and polyunsaturated fats. These fats are often liquid, such as olive oil and vegetable oil.

How to Eat

It's not just what you eat that matters, it's also how you eat. Mindful eating encourages you to pay attention to what you're eating. As a result, you're likely to eat less and enjoy it more.

Here are some tips for developing better eating habits.

- **Eat slowly.** A study published in the Journal of Clinical Endocrinology & Metabolism says that eating a meal quickly curtails the release of hormones in the gut that make you feel full. Eating fast doesn't give the stomach enough time to signal the brain that you're full. Next thing you know, you've overeaten and feel heavy, bloated, and sleepy. Eat slowly and tune in to your body's signals. Don't eat when you're full. Spend a minimum of 15 minutes eating each meal, ideally 20 to 30 minutes.

- **Pay attention to your meal.** Are you talking, watching TV, reading, or driving while you eat? Are you agitated or anxious? Not paying attention can cause you to overeat. Try to relax and focus on what you are eating. Many people practice silence and/or offer prayers before eating. This also helps them to slow down and shifts their focus to the eating process.

- **Enjoy your food.** Become more aware of what your food tastes like. Use all of your senses to enjoy your food and the process of eating it—from the pleasant colors and aromas of the food on your plate to the taste in your mouth and the feeling of how it goes down your food pipe into your stomach.

- **Chew each bite thoroughly.** "The more you chew, the less you will weigh". Few years ago, we had a dinner with a friend who was fairly thin. When asked about the secret of his weight, he told us that he chews each bite 32 times— that's it. He doesn't curtail his diet or exercise fanatically. I thought WOW. This reminded me of a science project I had done in high school where I tested if obesity is related to the speed of eating. I have since advised a number of my patients, and colleagues to chew thoroughly. It has worked for quite a few of them. Try it. This is an amazing tip that can work for anyone. Experts suggest chewing each bite 8 to 32 times. Make a small commitment to do so with your next major meal. Keep practicing until it becomes habit. Don't be afraid to chew till you start "drinking your solids and eating your liquids".

Food for Thought

It takes about 100 ears of corn to process one cup of corn oil. If you eat three pieces of fried chicken, you are getting about one-quarter cup of oil. Did nature intend for you to consume 25 ears of corn in one sitting?

When to Eat

People eat for many reasons: boredom, anxiety, stress, socialization, and, sometimes, hunger. Too often in our society, we don't pay attention to our hunger signals. Instead, we eat for other reasons, and quite often that results in eating too often and too much. Here are some ideas for controlling when you eat.

> **Did You Know?**
> The average consumption of calories in the United States is 3,800 calories per day.

- **Eat when you're hungry.** Wait for the hunger pangs before you eat. If your stomach is rumbling and you genuinely feel hungry, go for the food. Sometimes it pays to stall—have a glass of water or distract yourself with another task and see if you're still hungry a few minutes later. Don't eat just because the clock says it's time. Studies of childhood obesity reveal that feeding infants on demand (when they cry to signal hunger) may result in healthier children than feeding them on a schedule. The same applies to adults "eat when you are hungry, not by the clock"
- **Create space between the meals.** Science has revealed that it takes more than four hours to empty the stomach. Therefore, one should wait for 4 hours or longer after the last meal. At the same time, it takes an average of 4 hours or longer to fill the bladder and have an urge to seek a urinal or bathroom. It is no wonder that Travel Centers of America have food joints and rest rooms packed together and spaced 3 hours or longer on major US highways.
- **Limit the number of meals per day.** In the old days, in most agrarian societies, majority of the people ate 2 meals a day, typically at 10 am and 6pm and occasional light snacks in early morning hours or the evening. There is an old quote that means: Those who eat three times a day are rogi (unhealthy); those who eat two times a day are bhogi (worldly); and those who eat once a day are yogi. I agree we aren't yogis, but two full meals a day plus small snacks or juice as necessary should be enough for most of us. The easiest way to start would be to replace your breakfast or lunch with light fruit.

How do I lose weight?

If you want to lose weight, the first thing you need to do is figure out how many calories you need to consume each day, balanced with how much exercise you do to burn off calories.

Your caloric needs will vary, depending on your weight, your metabolism, and your level of activity.

But there is a simple formula for determining how many calories an average person needs. Just add a zero to the end of your desired weight in pounds, and that is the number of calories you need.

For example, if you want to weigh 150 pounds, you need 1,500 calories a day.

The maximum recommended is 2,000 calories. Unfortunately, most people in the United States consume far more than that and thus the obesity epidemic. Remember, a healthy weight is good for your heart!

Researchers have completed thousands of studies on weight loss, and authors have written even more books on the topic. Yet, there are few hard and fast rules on weight loss, other than you should eat a healthy diet that has fewer calories than you burn each day. No one diet plan is right for everyone, but here are some tips that may help you lose weight and not gain it back.

Classification of Overweight and Obesity by BMI, Waist Circumference, and Associated Disease Risks

Disease Risk* Relative to Normal Weight and Waist Circumference

	BMI
Underweight	<18.5
Normal	18.5–24.9
Overweight	25.0–29.9
Obesity	30.0–34.9
	35.0–39.9
Extreme Obesity	40.0+

Source: http://www.nhlbi.nih.gov/health/public/heart/obesity/lose_wt/bmi_dis.htm

Body Mass Index Table To use the table, find your height in the left column. Then move across to your weight. The number at the top of the column is your BMI.

BMI	19	20	21	22	23	24	25	26	27	28	29	30	31	32	33	34	35
Height (inches)	Body Weight (pounds)																
58	91	96	100	105	110	115	119	124	129	134	138	143	148	153	158	162	167
59	94	99	104	109	114	119	124	128	133	138	143	148	153	158	163	168	173
60	97	102	107	112	118	123	128	133	138	143	148	153	158	163	168	174	179
61	100	106	111	116	122	127	132	137	143	148	153	158	164	169	174	180	185
62	104	109	115	120	126	131	136	142	147	153	158	164	169	175	180	186	191
63	107	113	118	124	130	135	141	146	152	158	163	169	175	180	186	191	197
64	110	116	122	128	134	140	145	151	157	163	169	174	180	186	192	197	204
65	114	120	126	132	138	144	150	156	162	168	174	180	186	192	198	204	210
66	118	124	130	136	142	148	155	161	167	173	179	186	192	198	204	210	216
67	121	127	134	140	146	153	159	166	172	178	185	191	198	204	211	217	223
68	125	131	138	144	151	158	164	171	177	184	190	197	203	210	216	223	230
69	128	135	142	149	155	162	169	176	182	189	196	203	209	216	223	230	236
70	132	139	146	153	160	167	174	181	188	195	202	209	216	222	229	236	243
71	136	143	150	157	165	172	179	186	193	200	208	215	222	229	236	243	250
72	140	147	154	162	169	177	184	191	199	206	213	221	228	235	242	250	258
73	144	151	159	166	174	182	189	197	204	212	219	227	235	242	250	257	265
74	148	155	163	171	179	186	194	202	210	218	225	233	241	249	256	264	272
75	152	160	168	176	184	192	200	208	216	224	232	240	248	256	264	272	279
76	156	164	172	180	189	197	205	213	221	230	238	246	254	263	271	279	287

Source: http://www.nhlbi.nih.gov/guidelines/obesity/bmi_tbl.htm

A. Make a Decision:
- Know your ideal body weight. Ask yourself what your ideal body weight is. Write it down. Many people do not know what their ideal body weight should be.

    Here's a formula to help you figure your ideal body weight (IBW):

    Men: 105 pounds, plus 6 pounds per inch over 5 feet. Women: 100 pounds, plus 5 pounds per inch over 5 feet. For example, if a man is 5 feet 10 inches tall, then his IBW would be 100 plus 7 times 10, which equals 170 pounds.

    Knowing your ideal weight may convince you to make the decision to lose weight. You can also calculate your body mass index to see where you stand.

    Are you normal weight, overweight, or obese? See table on page 45.

    Use the tables that follow to determine your BMI and estimate your coronary artery disease risk based on your BMI and waist circumference.

- Ask yourself the tough question: Do I really need to lose weight? You may think the obvious answer is yes, but it's more complicated than that. Self-help author and motivational speaker Tony Robbins says, "It is in moments of decision that our destiny is shaped." If you make a decision to lose weight, nothing can stop you, but many people never make that decision because they are not 100 percent certain. They may have too much pain linked to losing weight. Once you make the decision to lose weight no matter what, that pain goes away. Too much weight is no longer a possibility in your life. You can make that decision when you have intellectual certainty [IC] as to why it is important to lose weight. Simply having a sincere desire does not cut it. Without that intellectual certainty (IC), we won't have the energy to sustain our efforts during rough times.

- Become aware. Most people underestimate how much food they eat. In a study published in 1992 in the New England Journal of Medicine, 47 percent of participants underestimated their food intake and 51 percent overestimated their exercise.

    Improve your ability to clearly see how much you eat and exercise. Keeping a journal, either online or on paper, often helps. However you choose to track it, try to bring awareness to your unconscious habits. As has been oft quoted, "We forget those things that we do not want to remember." We may not want to remember that we are overweight so we forget and let loose at meal-times.

B. Choose Right Foods:
- Choose foods that fill you up, not fatten you up. The 2010 Dietary Guidelines for Americans suggests eating more foods that are high in water and/or dietary fiber. These foods typically have fewer calories per gram, also referred to as low calorie density foods. High-fat foods have a higher calorie density. For a healthy diet that fills you up and supplies necessary nutrients, eat plenty of vegetables, fruit, and dietary fiber. Lower your intake of high-fat and sugary foods. Sugary foods are notorious for providing lots of calories but not filling you up—at least not for long. They also disturb your sugar level, make you hungry and create addiction. Evidence shows that eating a diet with low calorie density foods improves weight loss and weight maintenance. Follow tips above about what to eat and how to improve the quality of foods you eat.

C. Reduce Your Hunger:
- Avoid appetizers and appetite stimulants. Limit things that will stimulate your hunger and make you eat more than you need. These include added salt, sugar, and fats. These additives are bad for your body and increase your risk of diseases such as obesity, diabetes and hypertension. Visual cues and smells may also make your mouth water, so steer clear of them when possible.

Remember not to order the cookies, the drinks and the chips when you are paying for the healthy sandwich at the SUBWAY checkout counter. Also avoid the temptation to order desserts after you have had a good meal.

- Tap into your alternate energy sources. Food is not the only source that provides us with energy. Deep breathing exercises, relaxation practices, stress management techniques, and adequate sleep are also important sources that charge our battery and provide us with sources of energy. The energy boost from these sources will automatically reduce the amount of food you need to eat. Self-help author Tony Robbins recommends taking 10 deep breaths three times a day and whenever you feel hungry. Start tapping into these vital resources of energy and watch the results.

- Meditate every day. Set aside 20 minutes a day to settle your mind and sharpen your awareness. Dr. R. Nagarathna, chief of yoga therapy at one of the premier yoga universities of the world, once told me, "Let us view obesity as the jitteriness of the mind and not a problem of food." As you settle your mind, the desire for excess food diminishes automatically. Meditation will also sharpen your sense of awareness of how much you have eaten. It will enable you to detect overeating before you feel bloated thereby breaking the vicious cycle of overeating.

You will be amazed how it will bless you in many ways and improve your sleep, efficiency, peak performance, relationships, and above all happiness.

D. Track your results:

- Hop on the scale. Experts disagree on how often you should weigh yourself—opinions range from twice a day to never. I'm an advocate for frequent weigh-ins. Place a sheet of paper in front of your scale and record your body weight at the same time every day; most people prefer to do it in the morning. It will become a daily reminder for you to know how much to eat today. Before you start your day, you will have an awareness of how much to eat all day. Are you on the right track? It will also show you the effects of travel and/or parties, so you can scale back before it goes out of hand.

- Maintain a 'Daily Reflections' diary. Spend two minutes a day keeping a food diary. If you think it will help keep you on track, you may also record your daily exercise. Here are some things to include:
  - What did I eat today? Be honest and include everything.
  - How did I feel while eating? Was I stressed, anxious, peaceful, calm, excited, or bored?
  - Did I chew well?
  - Did I stick to my decision to eat healthy?

After you finish writing, close your eyes and reflect for two minutes about what you ate and whether you followed your commitments, again, awareness is important. Most people don't eat as healthy as they think. Just by becoming aware, you can create big changes. It works like magic.

E. Other things you can do.

- Read about nutrition. Reinforce the knowledge you already have and increase your understanding of healthy eating. Subscribe to magazines, read books like this, read the health section of your newspaper, or search for information on the Internet.

- Share your knowledge. If you start teaching others how to lose weight, you may lose more weight in the process. Again, it goes back to awareness and commitment to your decision. In his book, 7 habits of Highly Effective people, Steven Covey says: "learn it, teach it and practice it". The same has worked successfully for years for groups like Alcoholic Anonymous etc.

- Find a support system. Studies show that the most successful diets are ones that involve support. Attending support group meetings is an effective way of keeping you motivated and on track.

Online support groups can also help and encourage you to stick to your goals. If you don't want to join a group, enlist a friend or family member to be your weight loss buddy — someone who can celebrate your successes and support your efforts. It goes without saying: " You are known by the company you keep"

- Visit your doctor. Stepping on the scales at your doctor's office may be all the incentive you need to get serious about losing weight. Talk to your doctor about your commitment to lose weight, and discuss what would be a good weight-loss plan for you. Your doctor can give you nutritional information and may refer you to a dietitian. Your health care team will reinforce your positive habits.

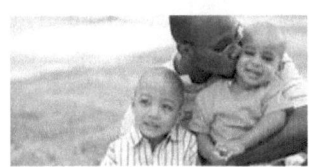

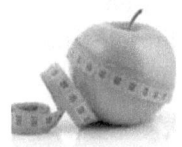

F. What not to do:

- Avoid Fad Diets. Do not start a diet that seems unnatural- eg. carbs only, protein only, fats only, liquids only diets. Trust your gut feeling: "If it smells wrong, it is probably wrong". When on a diet, watch out for any side effects. If symptoms of nausea, stomach pains, sleep disturbances etc. remain persistent, something is probably wrong and your new diet may be interfering with your metabolism. After the first 30 days, the right diet should make you feel better and more energetic. The right diet should also reduce hunger on its own. If you continue to remain hungry after the first 30 days, the diet may not be right for you and it is not likely to work.

- Don't overdo it. Do not expect results faster than losing one pound per week. Remember "slow and steady wins the race". Finally, avoid being the first on the bus for a new diet no matter how promising it seems. Majority of new diets have proven to be fads over the last 50+ years. When in doubt, follow common sense and come closer to nature. Listen to your body and your mind and you will be on the path to right foods and right weight. When it comes to food, weight, blood sugar or blood pressure, remember "Less is more".

Get Active: How to Do It

If you're like most Americans, you don't think you have the time or energy to work out. You, my friend, are a classic couch potato. But it's time to get moving! Inactivity is a huge risk factor for coronary artery disease. Now, that doesn't mean you have to start running marathons to reduce your risk. Simply getting more activity into your daily life can make a big difference.

That's because regular exercise strengthens your heart muscle (remember, the heart *is* a muscle) and the rest of your cardiovascular system. It also increases the number of *capillaries*, or small blood vessels that carry oxygen and nutrients to your body's cells, improving your circulation and reducing blood pressure. In addition, exercise increases the ability of the *mitochondria*, the "power plants" within your cells, to produce energy, making it easier for your body to use insulin and reducing your risk of diabetes. And by creating more muscle, it creates more muscle cells, which, next to your brain, are your body's biggest users of glucose.

A key benefit of exercise, of course, is that it burns calories, helping you lose excess body fat and maintain a healthy weight. Regular exercise also helps reduce central obesity, that "visceral" fat we discussed earlier, increases levels of HDL, or good cholesterol, and helps reduce blood pressure.

There are emotional benefits to exercise as well. Staying fit helps reduce feelings of depression and anxiety, improves your mood, and promotes a sense of well-being. Plus, regular physical activity strengthens muscles, bones, and joints, and reduces your risk of some forms of cancer.

Activity	Calories (per minute)
Sleep	0.5
Reading	1.5
Eating	2
Driving	2
Standing	2
Slow Walking	3 to 4
Casual Walking	4 to 5
Fast Walking	6 to 8
Jogging	7 to 9
Running	10 to 12

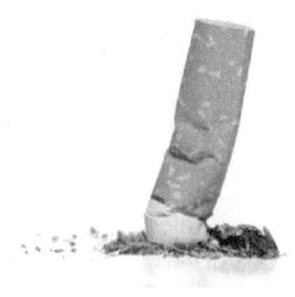

If you're already in good health, you can start an exercise program any time. But if you have questions, talk to us. If you've had a heart attack or stroke, we may want you to exercise under medical supervision. Also, if you've had chest pain or discomfort in the last month, if you tend to lose consciousness or fall because of dizziness, feel extremely out of breath after even mild exertion (such as walking a short distance), or are already taking medications for high blood pressure or coronary artery disease, we may recommend very gentle exercise.

If we've given you the go-ahead to exercise, start gradually. If you feel dizzy or faint or have chest pain or any other uncomfortable symptoms, let us know immediately. Dr. Kumar may want to conduct a *stress test* to check the condition of your heart before you begin working out.

Getting Started

The best way to get started with exercising is slowly. Nice and easy. Even a brief 5- to 10-minute walk is better than nothing.

There are three basic types of exercises: those that increase your body's flexibility, such as stretching or *yoga*; those that strengthen your body's muscular and skeletal system, such as weight lifting and strength-training exercises; and those that strengthen your cardiovascular and pulmonary system, such as brisk walking, bicycling, or swimming.

To reduce your risk of coronary artery disease, focus on aerobic exercise. This includes activities that can be done continuously using the large muscles in your legs, forcing your heart to work harder than normal. Over time, this strengthens your heart, increasing its efficiency even when you're not exercising. Good aerobic activities include brisk walking, jogging, bicycling, dancing, swimming, and cross-country skiing.

Use the "talk test" to measure your exercise intensity. You should be able to talk with a little effort as you're exercising. If you can't carry on a conversation at all, you're working too hard. But if you can speak easily, or even sing, you need to work a bit harder. This appropriate rate of exertion is considered "moderate-intensity" exercise. As you get fitter, you can challenge yourself to more vigorous exercise, gradually forcing your body to work harder.

You don't have to hit the gym or the treadmill to get moving Lifestyle activities like gardening, housework, walking your dog, and yard work "count" as physical activity. So do hobbies that get you off the couch, such as golf (skip the cart), bowling, and even window shopping! Focus on activities you enjoy and can continue for a lifetime and you'll find that getting fit is easier and more fun than you ever thought.

Snuff the Cigarette

If you are one of the estimated 45 million adults who smoke cigarettes, you are significantly increasing your chances of heart disease. In fact, a smoker's risk of developing coronary heart disease is two to four times higher than that of a nonsmoker. And it's not just heart disease you're courting. According to the Centers for Disease Control and Prevention, about 8.6 million people in the United States have at least one serious illness caused by smoking.

Smoking cigarettes releases toxins into the blood that contribute to *atherosclerosis*. As you may recall from Chapter 4, atherosclerosis occurs when the arteries leading to the heart become clogged with *plaque* or damaged with scars on the artery wall, narrowing the passageway through which blood can flow.

Smoking also reduces your heart's ability to pump blood. In one study, scientists studied ultrasound images of the hearts of smokers and nonsmokers between ages 20 and 40. Even after a two-hour break from cigarettes, the smokers had significantly weaker *left ventricles*, the part of the heart that pumps oxygen-rich blood to most of your body. This decreased pumping ability causes extra strain on the heart, weakening valves and stressing the heart muscle, all of which increases the risk of heart attack and stroke.

The Benefits of Quitting

Quitting smoking has significant short- and long-term benefits, both for reducing your risk of heart disease and improving your overall health. Within 20 minutes of quitting, your heart rate and blood pressure drop. Within one year, your risk of coronary artery disease has been halved, and within five years, your risk of stroke is the same as that of a nonsmoker.

There are several ways to quit smoking but none are "easy" or "foolproof." Plus, it may take you several tries before you really stop smoking forever.

One option—which I don't recommend—is to go "cold turkey" and just stop smoking one day. You're better off, however, working with Dr. Kumar or another doctor. He can prescribe medications shown to improve smoking cessation success; point you to nicotine replacement products like gum, sprays, or patches that can help wean you from the addiction of nicotine; and recommend support groups. For instance, Zyban (bupropion), an FDA-approved antidepressant, and Chantix (varenicline) each affect chemicals in the brain that keep you addicted to nicotine. They reduce the feeling of pleasure associated with smoking by attaching to nicotine receptors in the brain; several studies find they can more than double your chances of successfully quitting.

The following can also help:

- **Decide on a purpose.** Are you quitting for your health? To see your kids grow up? To save money? All of the above?
- **Set a quit date.** This is your deadline for quitting. On this date, you will smoke your last cigarette. Make sure everyone around you knows your quit date so they can be supportive.
- **Clean up your environment.** Throw away all tobacco products, lighters, and ashtrays to physically rid you of the habit. You know what they say: out of sight, out of mind.
- **Seek support.** Whether it's your friends, family, me, a counselor, coworkers, or a support group, having people you can talk to who understand your struggle will help you stay strong. Many hospitals and health centers offer free hotlines and meetings. You can also find help online. Start at the American Lung Association at *www.lungusa.org*.
- Identify and avoid your smoking triggers. Stress, certain foods or drink, and certain environments in which you regularly smoked (like a bar) can create that urge. To avoid caving, avoid those situations or places. For instance, if you typically have a cigarette with a cup of coffee every morning, switch to tea. If you usually smoke when you drink, stop drinking. Or only have a drink in nonsmoking environments.

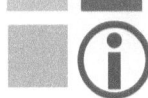

Did you know?

The United States Department of Health and Human Services provides a five-day countdown to quitting smoking to get you through the first and hardest part of quitting. You can find it at: www.surgeongeneral.gov/tobacco/5daybook.htm. Or check out http://www.surgeongeneral.gov/tobacco/ for a huge list of resources to help you quit.

Get Rid of the Stress — Get Rid of the Risk

Stress has long been known to have negative effects on your heart and the rest of your body. Stress stems from the age old "fight-or-flight" response. When you're faced with a threat—whether a car accident or a deadline at work—your body produces hormones such as cortisol that make your heart pump faster and more forcefully, signal your muscles to respond quickly, and help you defend yourself or flee the situation. However, too much stress—particularly constant, unrelenting stress (also known as chronic stress)—can raise blood pressure and cause a systemic inflammatory response, increasing your risk of coronary artery disease. It may also increase that visceral fat around your middle.

In addition, if you already have heart disease, stress may raise your risk of dying from it. One small study from the American College of Cardiology and the University of Florida found that people with coronary artery disease who experience significant stress can develop *ischemia*, or restriction in blood flow to parts of the heart. In addition, the study found those who develop ischemia are three times more likely to die in the next five years than people with coronary artery disease who are better at managing their day-to-day stress.

That sounds scary, doesn't it? But stress in your life isn't fatal—in fact, all of us deal with it continually. The trick is learning how to manage it so it doesn't manage you.

> *"If you want to live longer, breathe slowly."*
> — Vinod Kumar, M.D., F.A.C.C.

Understanding Stress

Stress is not harmful because of the stressful trigger itself but because of your response to it. While you may not be able to change the stressful event, you can control how you respond to it. For instance, when you're stuck in traffic, you can choose to get all upset and pound the steering wheel and complain—or listen to soothing music or simply enjoy having some time alone.

The key is to learn and practice stress management techniques.

Try these tips:

- **Breathe.** Take time each day to breathe deeply while concentrating on a positive mental image. Take deep breaths, letting your belly expand on the inhale and recede on the exhale.

Imagine breathing in relaxation and breathing out worries. When you feel your attention wander, gently return your focus to your breathing. When you're under stress, taking a five minute breathing break a couple times a day can make a big difference compared to letting the stress accumulate. Deep breathing allows you to relax, focus, and center yourself to handle the stress along the way. In fact, scientific evidence shows that creatures with a slower breathing rate live longer than those who breathe faster. The following chart shows the differences in lifespan in direct proportion to breathing rate.

Breaths per minute		Average life in years
Mouse	300	1
Rabbit	70	8
Monkey	32	10
Frog	25	20
Man	12	100
Snake	7	150-250
Turtle	1	300-500

- **Get off the couch.** Physical activity reduces anxiety and lets you work out feelings of anger and aggression, reducing levels of inflammatory, stress related hormones.
- **Let go.** Accept that not everything is in your control. Talk out your troubles with someone you love, a spiritual adviser, or a therapist, and focus on those aspects of your life you can change.
- **Exercise your mind.** Pick up a relaxation CD, which will direct you through a visualization exercise. Or create a visual image— a peaceful place where you feel calm—and take a few minutes to imagine yourself there. Listen to your favorite music, write in a journal, or take time to explore a favorite hobby regularly. Releasing your stress with such behaviors can help reduce it, ultimately reducing the added physical effects of stress, such as increased heart rate and high blood pressure.
- **Pray or meditate regularly.** Repeat a name or phrase, also called a mantra. Focusing on one word help quieten your mind. You can create your own mantra by using a favorite word or the name of someone you love. This type of mental vacation can significantly reduce the effects of stress on your body.

- **Let go.** Sometimes acknowledging that a higher power is in control can help you let go of things you can't control.
- **Maintain a healthy diet with lots of whole grains, fruits, and vegetables.** Eating well helps you feel better and provides the energy you need to get through the day. A poor diet only adds to your stress by making you fatigued and irritable, while a diet rich in nutrients and minerals boosts your immune system, helping it ward off stress related illnesses.
- **Make sleep a priority and aim for at least seven hours per night.** Your body needs a full night's rest to repair itself from the wear and tear of the day. Without this rest, it can't effectively fight stress.
- **Mentally scan your body.** Focus your attention on physical sensations like pain, tension, or relaxation in different parts of your body. Imagine drawing heat or relaxation to these parts of your body with your breath. Or contract and release one muscle at a time throughout your body. These systematic exercises relax your muscles and moderate your breathing, reducing the effects of stress on your body.

> *"Learn to manage stress so it doesn't manage you."*
> — Ashish Gupta, M.D.

Yoga and Meditation

Yoga and *meditation* originated in India, where they have been practiced for thousands of years. Both are "mind/body" techniques designed to induce a feeling of relaxation and serenity many people lack in their day-to-day lives.

Yoga involves focusing on precise movements and poses based on balance, concentration, and breath control. While there are many schools or types of yoga, the main principle is the same:

Controlling your breathing can help you gain control of your body and mind.

Meditation is a practice that lets you connect your body with your mind. It allows you to develop awareness of your internal state, an integral step in reducing stress. When meditating, you must first be aware of the onset of a stressful reaction or effect before you can prevent the resulting harmful, physiological responses that may lead to disease.

One government funded study found that heart patients who studied transcendental meditation (the type with a mantra) showed slight improvement in insulin levels and significant reduction in systolic and diastolic blood pressure.

Another study of heart patients and healthy participants found that six weeks of a 90 minute yoga and meditation session three times a week, plus home practice, reduced blood pressure, heart rate, and body mass index.

A study by Duke University Medical Center's Department of Psychiatry found that people who practiced mantra based meditation for one hour for four meetings and practiced at home 15 to 20 minutes twice a day significantly reduced their levels of perceived stress and improved their moods.

The evidence is clear: yoga and meditation can significantly reduce your stress and help you maintain a heart healthy lifestyle day to day.

So start practicing!

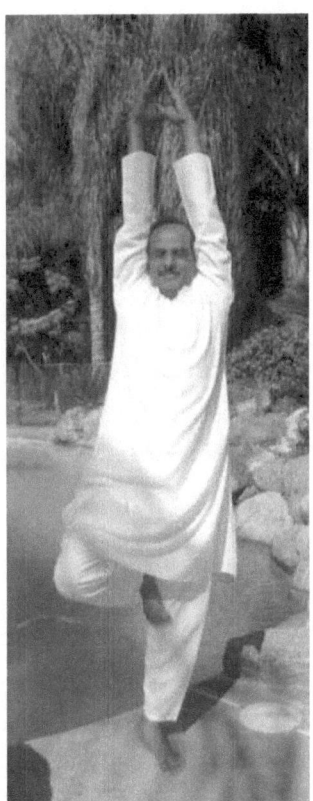

Good Family, Good Heart

One way to get the "fabulous four" in an integrated manner is to participate in our wellness program to prevent and reverse heart disease: Good Family, Good Heart.

This one-day workshop emphasizes an individual's modifiable risk factors for heart related illness. During the workshop, myself and Dr. Kumar highlight the lifestyle choices you can change to protect your heart and allow you to live a longer, fuller life. Through this program, you learn about diet and nutrition, exercise and fitness, stress reduction techniques and how to garner support from those around you.

We begin our full day workshop with an introductory lecture on the heart. Dr. Kumar present information on the structure of the heart, cardiovascular diseases, diagnosis, cardiological testing, common surgical procedures, and risk factors. He even dissect a sheep heart and allow each participant to touch the heart muscle and take a closer look at just how tiny an artery really is. We believe this hands on approach to heart-health education provides an exciting and enriching environment that helps strengthen the relationship between doctor, patient, and self.

During the diet and nutrition portions of the program we discuss, naturally, food. I teach you how to accurately read a nutrition label and encourage you to apply that skill every day until it becomes second nature. We also provide breakfast and lunch and discuss the nutritional elements of the healthy foods you're eating using an applied learning technique.

Next we discuss fitness and exercise. You learn how to add more aerobic activity to your daily routine and how to get the most out of any activity. I also teach you some simple exercises that you can do at home or at the office without purchasing any special equipment. Weather permitting, we enjoy a brisk nature walk together. The message of this section of the workshop is that you must exercise to keep your heart muscle fit and healthy.

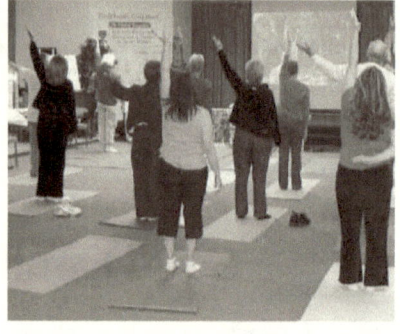

An often overlooked risk factor for heart disease is stress. We all must have a certain level of stress in our lives; it's nature's way of protecting us. Should we ever be approached by a lion, our body must gear up for the fight that may ensue or be prepared to run as fast as possible to escape the situation. This is often referred to as your body's "fight or flight" response. The problem with stress levels today is that we have an ever increasing pace of life and often have very little control over what is happening to us.

This increases our stress reaction and puts additional strain on our hearts. This stress can manifest itself as high blood pressure, overeating, or depression. All of these take their toll on your body and specifically, your heart.

During the workshop, I show you several scientifically proven methods of stress reduction, including deep breathing techniques like those practiced in yoga. You enjoy an hour long yoga session with an emphasis on pranayamas, or deep breathing, exercises. These exercises lower heart rate and blood pressure, not to mention providing deep relaxation. Deep breathing is a wonderful way to relax your body from the inside out.

Finally, we discuss the importance of support. After struggling with a name for my program, we decided on Good Family, Good Heart. We chose this name because we believe that family, friends, and loved ones are the backbone of your success. Those we share our lives with have a direct impact on the activities we participate in, the foods we eat, and the lifestyle we lead. We encourage everyone who chooses to attend a Good Family, Good Heart Wellness Program to bring a loved one with them. Together, we can overcome these lifestyle hang-ups that are ailing our hearts.

 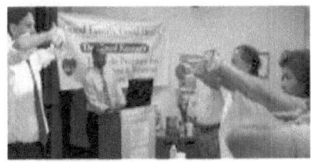 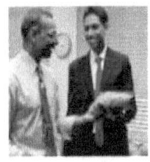 

My hope is that each person who attends one of our events decides to take part in our monthly support group meetings. I want each of you to feel as though the others who have attended are your extended family. As the program continues and grows, so will your extended family.

The bottom line is this: Children today suffer from obesity, diabetes, and other health concerns that increase their risk for heart disease. We can work together to teach our children to live healthier lives, to make wiser choices, and to be happier. It is your responsibility to ensure the success of the next generation; they are counting on you to pass on the traits and skills they will need to make a happy life for themselves someday. We can lead by example, as we know is always best. We can stop this cycle of disease and death. We can overcome this epidemic, one person at a time.

> "Please join us in leaving a positive trail of footprints for our children to walk upon, so that everyone can enjoy the blessings of a good family and good heart."

Test Your Knowledge

Answer the following questions to see how much you have learned about eating and heart health. Then turn to the next page for the correct answers.

1. **What health problems can be affected by obesity?**
    a. Heart attack, stroke, and other cardiovascular disease
    b. Diabetes
    c. Certain cancers, including colon, kidney, and breast
    d. All of the above

2. **What foods should I eat the most for a heart-healthy diet?**
    a. Fresh fruits and vegetables
    b. Red meats
    c. Desserts
    d. Prepackaged meals

3. **What foods should I limit for a heart-healthy diet?**
    a. Whole-grains
    b. Low-fat dairy
    c. Salts, sugars, and fats
    d. Fruits

4. **All of the following are good habits for mindful eating except:**
    a. Eat slowly
    b. Watch TV
    c. Chew thoroughly
    d. Pay attention to your meal

5. **All of the following can reduce your hunger except:**
    a. Meditation
    b. Deep breathing exercises
    c. Relaxation techniques
    d. Avoiding salt, sugar and fats
    e. All of the above

6. **Exercise improves all of the following except:**
    a. Number of capillaries
    b. Ability of mitochondria to produce energy
    c. Heart rhythm
    d. Weight

   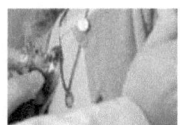

7. The best exercise for your heart is:
   a. Aerobic
   b. Strength training
   c. Flexibility
   d. Yoga

8. Chronic stress leads to heart disease by:
   a. Increasing blood pressure
   b. Restricting blood flow
   c. Increasing inflammation
   d. All of the above

Answers:
1. d 2. a 3. c 4. b 5. e d 6. c 7. a 8. d

It's a Family Affair

Family history of heart disease puts you at higher risk of developing heart attack.

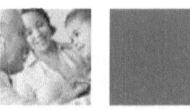
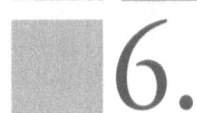

6.

We can't choose our family—which also means we can't choose our family medical history. That means if you have a history of heart disease in your family, you must be extra vigilant about controlling other risk factors. It also means that your children may have an increased risk. So by focusing on your own health, you are also focusing on the health of your entire family.

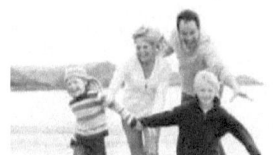

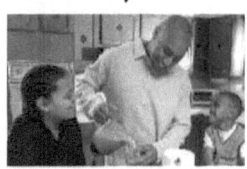

Family History Factors That Raise Your Risk of Heart Disease

The red flags to watch for are a diagnosis of heart disease in your mother or sister before age 65 or in your father or brother before age 55. You may also have a higher risk if your grandparents, aunts, or uncles were diagnosed with heart disease before those ages. If you're not 100 percent sure about your family history, speak up!

The best way to find out is to ask your relatives. Ask about any major medical conditions your relatives had, how old they were when they were diagnosed, how they died, and how old they were when they died. Pay attention to what your relatives say. They may be talking about "tired blood," which could be a sign of *congestive heart failure*. Or "blew an artery," which could be a stroke. Or "high sugar," which could mean diabetes.

Also ask about your family's ethnic background because certain ethnicities are at a higher risk for developing *coronary artery disease*, such as African Americans, Mexican Americans, American Indians, native Hawaiians, and some Asian Americans. There is no dumb question—play it safe and cover all your bases with relatives in the know because this history may impact the rest of your life as well as your children's (and grandchildren's) lives. You can also use the U.S. Surgeon General's Family History Initiative to help you map out your personal family health history. It's available at http://www.hhs.gov/familyhistory/.

Your family history is one of the most helpful tools when it comes to predicting your risk of heart conditions and planning the most effective way to reduce that risk.

Better yet, knowing your family history and making lifestyle changes as a result doesn't just benefit your health. It also means you're passing on a healthier history to your children and grandchildren. Even if you can't change the health histories of older relatives, you can be a great role model for everyone in your family by inspiring them to lead a healthier lifestyle through your example.

Getting Your Family Involved

When you live in a family, that family lives a certain kind of lifestyle together—whether healthy or unhealthy. Research finds that one cause of an unhealthy family history is that families often share habits that increase their risk factors, such as a sedentary lifestyle and unhealthy diet. So if you're serious about improving your heart health, you've got to include the whole family.

Of course, this may be easier said than done. It might be difficult to convince your kids to give up a greasy fast food burger for a more healthful turkey burger, but if that's the only option offered for dinner, and everyone else in the family is eating it, they're more likely to make the switch.

Also, don't think of these changes as putting the family on a strict diet and military style exercise plan—think of them as manageable adjustments that will improve everyone's well being immediately.

Here are some simple changes the entire family can make.

- **Eat at least one meal a day together as a family.** If you serve healthful, delicious foods, your kids will learn better eating habits. In fact, studies show that family meals play an important role in promoting positive dietary intake in children, and that children in families who eat together regularly are less likely to be overweight.

- **Incorporate more fruits, vegetables, and whole grains into your family's meals.** For example, use whole wheat pasta, make meatballs with lean ground turkey instead of ground meat, and serve with marinara sauce plumped up with added veggies. Add a leafy green salad with chopped tomatoes, carrots, and peppers, and you have a delicious, filling, *healthy* dinner.

- **Don't smoke**—and encourage your kids not to pick up the habit. Offer to help anyone in your family who smokes to quit. And make your house and car no smoking zones.

- **Get active as a family.** Round up everyone to take a walk or bike ride after dinner, head out to the park to play Frisbee, to the pool to swim on weeknights and weekends, or sign up to help coach your child's sport team.
- **Encourage your kids to get off the couch, even if it means limiting television or computer time.** Just keep in mind that you're their first role model, so you need to set a good example. Join your kids in fun activities like playing basketball, dancing, and even hula-hooping. Your goal should be for everyone in your family to get at least 30 minutes of moderate activity every day.
- **Have healthy snacks**—like fresh fruit, low sugar and low-fat yogurt, sliced carrots and low-fat dip—on hand all the time. Stop buying junk food and soft drinks. And save treats like candy, cookies, and ice cream for special occasions.
- **Make it fun!** Ask your kids (or grandkids) what they'd like to do, and don't be afraid to try new activities. If your family members enjoy what they're doing, they're more likely to stick with it—and those healthy habits mean they'll be at lower risk for heart disease for the rest of their lives.

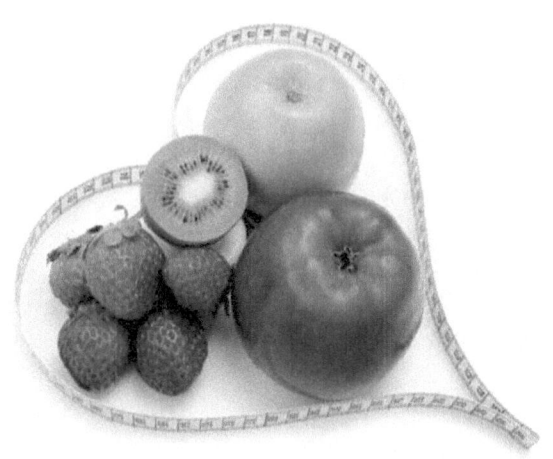

Test Your Knowledge

Answer the following questions to see how much you have learned about the link between family history and heart disease. Then turn to the next page for the correct answers.

1. Which of the following is a "red flag" for a history of heart disease in your family?
    a. Your father died from a heart attack at age 49.
    b. Your mother has breast cancer.
    c. Your 64-year-old, overweight brother has high cholesterol.
    d. Your grandfather died of unexplained causes.

2. One of the best ways you can get your kids to eat healthier is by:
    a. Choosing healthier items on the fast food menu
    b. Only eating out twice a week
    c. Eating at least one meal a day together as a family
    d. Buying 100-calorie snack packs

3. One of the best ways to get your kids more physically active is by:
    a. Buying them a treadmill
    b. Getting them a membership to the gym
    c. Doing physically active family activities together
    d. Hiring a personal trainer

4. The best example for healthy living for your kids is:
    a. You
    b. Healthy friends
    c. Joining a sports team
    d. Taking up running

Answers: 1.a 2.c 3.c 4.a

Time for a Test

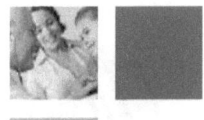
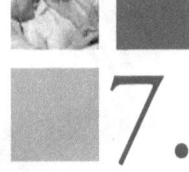

7.

Learning what the most commonly performed tests really mean.

So far, you've learned how your heart works, what *coronary artery disease* is, and the risk factors associated it. You've also calculated your own risk of a *heart attack* with the Framingham Risk Analysis. Now it's time to learn about the most commonly performed cardiovascular related tests, the tests that will help your doctor learn about any potential problems with your cardiovascular system. Most important, you'll learn what the results mean.

Electrocardiogram (EKG or ECG)

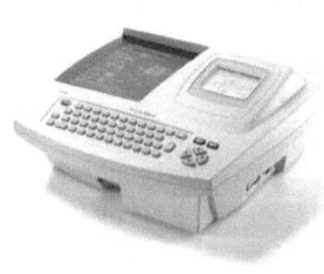

What is it? An *electrocardiogram*, also known as an EKG or ECG, checks for problems associated with the electrical function of your heart. Recall from Chapter 1 that an electrical signal beginning in your heart's *right atrium* and traveling to the bottom of the heart is responsible for every beat. An EKG simply measures the rate and regularity of your heart beat and the strength of your heart's electric signal.

Why is it conducted? An electrocardiogram is ordered to evaluate cardiac symptoms such as chest pain, *ischemia* (in which parts of the heart don't receive sufficient blood flow), or *palpitations*.

How is it conducted? During an EKG, 12 electrodes (soft, quarter-sized patches) are placed on different areas of your body (usually the chest, arms, and legs). Next, you lie still for a few minutes while the electrodes measure your heart's electrical signal, and a machine records the pattern on paper or displays it on a monitor. This is called a resting EKG.

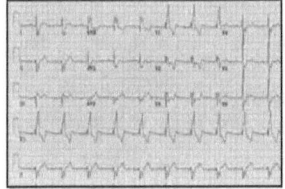
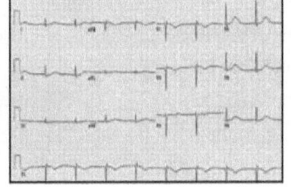
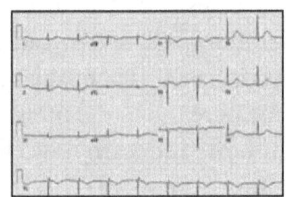

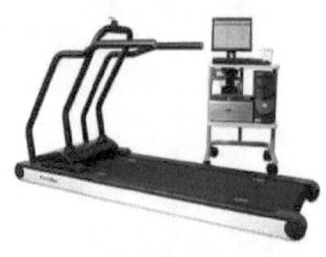

If, however, your heart has a problem that doesn't occur all the time, you may need a stress test or an ambulatory electrocardiography with a Holter monitor. A stress test is an EKG while you walk on a treadmill or ride a stationary bicycle. The activity makes your heart work harder, making it easier to diagnose certain conditions.

A Holter monitor is a recorder you wear for an extended period of time while you go about your normal activities. The monitor records your heart rhythm over time.

What do the results mean? An EKG is considered normal if your heart beats between 60 and 100 beats per minute (bpm) with a consistent and even rhythm. Abnormal results are any readings above or below the normal range, or results that show spikes or inconsistent rhythms.

Cardiac catheterization (angiogram)

What is it? A cardiac catheterization, or "cardiac cath," helps confirm whether you have heart disease and how bad it is, evaluates the function of your heart muscle, and determines whether you need additional treatment. It's often performed along with coronary angiography (see below.)

Why is it done? A cardiac catheterization checks for blocked arteries, which can lead to a heart attack and measures blood pressure within the heart and the amount of oxygen in your blood.

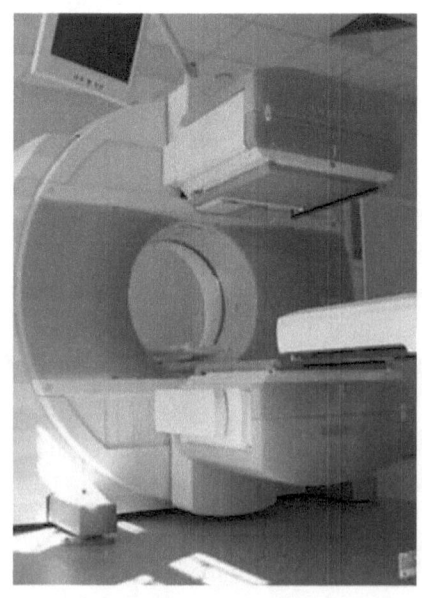

How is it done? This test is performed on an outpatient basis, often as part of a coronary angiography (described below). After a mild sedative and the insertion of an IV, a long thin, flexible tube called a *catheter* is inserted through a blood vessel in your arm, groin (upper thigh), or neck, and threaded through to your heart. That enables the doctor to measure the blood pressure within your heart and learn how efficiently it pumps.

Generally, the doctor threads the tube into your *coronary arteries* and then injects dye into your bloodstream. As the dye flows through your coronary arteries, special X-rays and movies are taken. You may need to hold your breath as the films are taken.

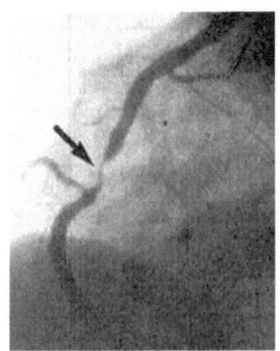

What do the results mean? The angiography is considered normal if it shows the dye flowing through the arteries evenly without any narrowing, blockage, or other discrepancies. Abnormal results show narrowing or blockage, possibly indicating a clot or aneurysm, or a growth or tumor growing against the artery.

Echocardiogram (transthoracic echocardiogram)

What is it? An *echocardiogram*, or *transthoracic echocardiogram* (TTE), is a test in which sound waves are used to depict the flow of blood through your heart.

Why is it conducted? It measures the effectiveness of your heart's valves and chambers. It is also used to evaluate heart murmurs and check how well your heart pumps blood to the rest of your body.

How is it performed? First, you get an EKG (as described earlier in this chapter). Then a gel is smoothed across your chest and a *transducer*—a device that produces high frequency sound—is placed on your ribs pointing toward the heart. The device "listens" to echoes of the sound from your heart and changes those echoes to electrical impulses. A machine then changes those impulses into a picture of your heart. Because your lungs or ribs can sometimes prevent the sound waves from going directly to the heart, a dye may be injected via an IV to create a clearer picture.

Another form of echocardiogram is called a *transesophageal echocardiogram* (TEE). In this procedure, the scope is inserted through your mouth and lowered down the esophagus to obtain the images. You'll be given medicine to help you relax, and the back of your mouth is numbed so you don't gag when the scope is inserted gently down your throat. The whole test takes about an hour, but you should plan on spending several hours at the doctor's office or hospital for preparation and monitoring after the test.

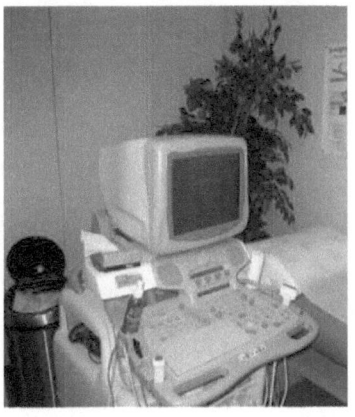

What do the results mean? Normal results show average sized chamber walls and valves that work without any leaking or narrowing. Additionally, your *ejection fraction*, or the amount of blood pumped out of the *left ventricle* with each heartbeat, should be more than 55 percent.

Abnormal results show large chambers or walls that are either thicker or thinner than normal, indicating poor blood flow or a previous heart attack. Leaky valves or an ejection fraction less than 55 percent also indicate a problem.

Magnetic resonance imaging (MRI)

What is it? A cardiovascular *magnetic resonance* imaging (MRI) uses strong magnets and radio waves to create a picture of the heart. It is often performed as part of a chest MRI.

Why is it conducted? MRI is used if an echocardiogram is inconclusive for coronary artery disease. It is less risky than *angiography* and can help pinpoint heart muscle damage.

How is it done? You lie on a table that moves into an imaging machine that looks like a large doughnut. A technician in the adjacent room observes and manages the test. In some cases, dye might be injected into your veins to make your heart show up on the image more clearly.

The cardiac MRI uses radio waves, magnets, and a computer to create three dimensional images of your heart as it beats, producing both still and moving pictures of your heart and major blood vessels. Some people feel claustrophobic inside an MRI machine, but newer "open MRI" models can help. Also, the machine makes loud humming and buzzing noises, so you can ask for earplugs if you want. It's important that you lie very still during the test, and you may have to hold your breath for 10 to 15 seconds when pictures are taken. The whole test takes about 45 to 90 minutes to perform, and you'll be monitored for some time afterward before you can leave.

> ### One Patient's Story
> *Chuck is a 26-year-old Bakersfield, California, resident with congestive heart failure. He's a rancher, and he knew something was wrong when he found he got out of breath just walking from the house to the barn—or when he'd run out of breath even while sitting still. When he came to me, I performed an echocardiogram that showed his heart was pumping at only 15 percent of its capacity. He began taking medication, and his ejection fraction improved.*

What do the results mean? The results depend on how your radiologist interprets them, but "abnormal" results can help identify heart valve disorders, heart abnormalities, or scarring of heart muscle.

Nuclear Scan

What is it?
A *nuclear heart scan* is a special kind of x-ray.

Why is it conducted?
It is used to look for any blockages.

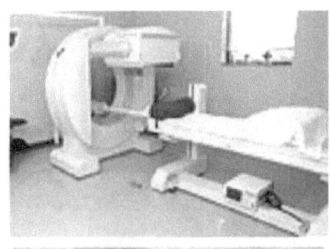

How is it done? A radioactive dye is injected into your bloodstream, and then images are taken to show the flow of blood through your heart and coronary arteries.

What do the results mean? The scan shows any problems with blood flow to and from the heart.

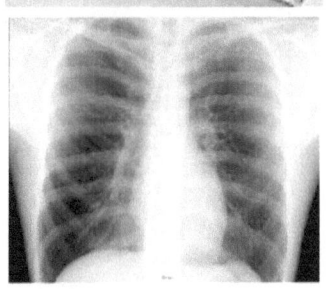

CT Angiogram

What is it? A *CT angiogram* is a minimally invasive test that provides a three dimensional image of your heart and blood vessels.

Why is it conducted? It helps diagnose blockages and/or *atherosclerosis*.

How is it done? You lie on the CT examination table, sometimes flat, sometimes on your side or stomach, depending on what is being reviewed. You have a small IV line inserted into your hand or arm, and a small dose of contrast material may be inserted through the IV. The scanner takes pictures as the material moves through your blood stream. You may need to hold your breath as each picture is taken.

What do the results mean? They can show any blockages or other problems with your coronary arteries or other blood vessels.

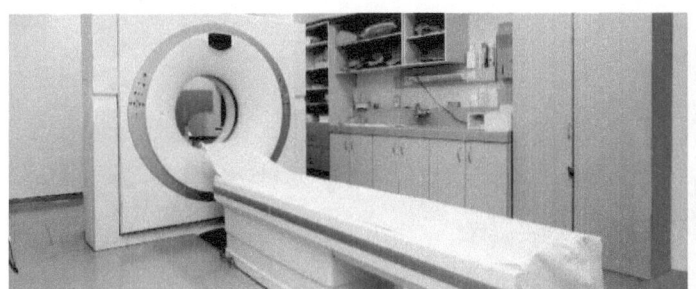
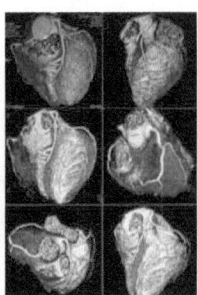

Test Your Knowledge

Answer the following questions to see how much you have learned about tests used to evaluate your cardiovascular health. Then turn to the next page for the correct answers.

1. Which test would be used to measure your heart's electrical signal?
    a. A cardiovascular MRI   b. A stress test
    c. An electrocardiogram   d. An ultrasound
2. If your doctor wanted to confirm heart disease and evaluate how bad it is, he or she might order a(n):
    a. Cardiac catheterization   b. MRI
    c. Echocardiogram   d. All of the above
3. Which test measures your ejection fraction?
    a. An MRI   b. An EKG
    c. A stress test   d. An echocardiogram
4. Cardiac catheterization is only performed on an inpatient basis since it is invasive.
    a. True   b. False

Answers: 1.c 2.d 3.d 4.b

Specific Conditions of the Heart

You know by now that the heart is a marvelously complex organ. Unfortunately, that complexity means that there are a variety of things that can go wrong with it. If you're diagnosed with a particular condition, learning as much about it as you can is the first step toward treating it.

Following is a brief explanation of eight common heart related conditions, along with their causes and treatment options. Keep in mind this is only an overview—we'll be happy to give more information to you about any of them.

Atherosclerosis and Heart Attacks

By age 40, 70% Americans already have evidence of plaque buildup in their arteries.

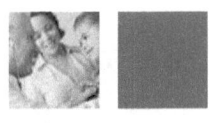
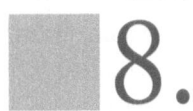

8.

Atherosclerosis occurs when fatty material, or *plaque*, collects along the walls of your arteries. The condition is a form of *arteriosclerosis*, in which the arteries thicken and harden with the plaque buildup. Meanwhile, what most people call a "*heart attack*," doctors call a "*myocardial infarction*," or MI. It occurs when the blood supply to the heart muscle, or *myocardium*, is drastically reduced or stopped.

Cause: Atherosclerosis occurs when fat, cholesterol, and other substances collect on artery walls and harden into plaque. Plaque makes arteries less flexible and affects blood flow. The plaque can also break off of the artery wall and fall into the bloodstream, creating a blockage and causing a heart attack or stroke.

The risk of atherosclerosis increases if you smoke; are obese; have diabetes, high blood cholesterol, or high blood pressure; follow a high fat diet; or have a family history of heart disease.

While the exact cause of atherosclerosis is unknown, we think it starts with damage to the *endothelium*, the innermost layer of the artery. Once this damage occurs, immune cells rush in to repair it, causing *inflammation* and increasing the buildup of plaque. As the plaque builds, the artery diameter decreases, restricting blood flow and oxygen supply to the rest of your body.

Angina, or chest pain, results from this reduced blood flow.

Symptoms: You may not have any symptoms from atherosclerosis until you have significant blockage and blood flow restriction. The primary symptoms are angina or leg pain (if the blocked artery is in the leg).

The pain of angina and a heart attack is usually described as pressure, tightness, heaviness, burning, indigestion, heartburn, or gas in the chest, or it may feel like someone is sitting on your chest.

These symptoms can also be felt in the arms, shoulders, neck, jaw, and throat, or in the back muscles. Angina might also lead to nausea, fatigue, weakness, palpitations, irregular heart beats, dizziness, a feeling of faintness, numbness in the arms, or excessive sweating. If you have these symptoms, pay attention to how long the pain lasts.

If it's more than a couple of minutes or medication doesn't improve it, call 911 and get to the closest emergency department immediately. You may be having a heart attack.

While some heart attacks are sudden and intense, most start with just a few mild symptoms. However, there are definite warning signs for heart attacks. They include chest discomfort, pain in other areas of the body, and shortness of breath. Women are more likely than men to experience nausea and light-headedness or to break out in a cold sweat.

Diagnosis: Diagnosis of atherosclerosis begins with a physical exam. When we listen to your heart, I'm listening for a *bruit*, an abnormal "whooshing" sound, and checking for a weak or absent pulse. We'll also check your cholesterol and blood sugar levels.

Tests commonly used in the diagnosis of atherosclerosis include an electrocardiogram, chest X-ray, *echocardiogram, angiography*, and *stress test*. Others include:

Ankle/brachial index. This test measures the blood pressure in your brachial artery (in your arm) and compares it to the blood pressure in your ankles. This test showsif the blood flow is consistent throughout your body.

C-reactive protein (CRP). This blood test measures a blood protein that shows the presence of inflammation. Levels of C-reactive protein are important because studies have shown that high levels of CRP consistently predicted recurrent coronary events in patients with unstable angina.

If doctors suspect you've had a heart attack, they will also order blood tests to check cardiac enzymes such as the troponin and creatine kinase enzymes (CK-MB). Levels of these enzymes increase a few hours after a heart attack begins.

Treatment:
As with all heart conditions, lifestyle changes like those described in Chapter 5 are key.

Medication:
You may also require clot-preventing drugs and medications to reduce your cholesterol and blood pressure, including:

- **Angiotensin–converting enzyme (ACE) inhibitors:** Commonly prescribed ACE inhibitors include captopril (Capoten), benazepril (Lotensin), and enalapril (Vasotec). These medications relax the blood vessels and prevent release of a hormone called *angiotensin II*, which causes blood vessels to narrow. Side effects may include cough, elevated blood potassium levels, low blood pressure, and dizziness.

- **Angiotensin II antagonists:** Valsartan (Diovan) and olmesartan (Benicar) are two commonly prescribed angiotensin antagonists. These drugs protect heart blood vessels from angiotensin II, which, in turn, helps widen the vessels. Side effects may include cough, low blood pressure, and drowsiness.
- **Antiplatelet agents.** These drugs prevent blood clots. They include medications like aspirin, dihydropyridine, and glycoprotein IIB/IIa inhibitors. All work to block the production of chemicals that enable clotting, such as thromboxane and *adenosine diphosphate*. Side effects include nausea, stomach ulcers, or *gastritis*.
- **Beta blockers.** This class of medication helps reduce your heart rate and cardiac output, which, in turn, lowers blood pressure. However, they are also used to treat cardiac *arrhythmias* and angina. Commonly prescribed beta blockers include atenolol (Tenormin) and betaxolol (Kerlone). Side effects include diarrhea, abdominal cramps, or nausea.
- *Calcium channel blockers.* These drugs prevent calcium from entering the muscle cells of the heart and arteries. This helps widen the arteries and reduce heart contractions. Common side effects may include constipation, low blood pressure, and nausea. Commonly prescribed calcium channel blockers include diltiazem (Cardizem), verapamil, amlodipine (Norvasc), nisoldipine (Sular), nifedipine (Adalat, Procardia), and nicardipine (Cardene).
- **Diuretics.** Medications in this class rid your body of excess fluids and sodium. They are also typically the first treatment tried for high blood pressure. They include chlorthalidone (Hygroton), furosemide (Lasix), hydrochlorothiazide (Esidrix), and triamterene (Dyrenium). Side effects may range from dehydration to blood chemistry abnormalities, such as potassium loss.
- **Statins.** Statins lower cholesterol levels by reducing the production of cholesterol in the liver. Commonly prescribed statins include atorvastatin (Lipitor), rosuvastatin (Crestor), fluvastatin (Lescol), and simvastatin (Zocor). Possible side effects include headache, nausea, vomiting, constipation, muscle aches, joint pain, and elevated liver enzymes.
- **Vasodilators.** Medications in this class dilate your blood vessels by relaxing their muscular walls. Nitroglycerin (Nitro-Bid, Nitro-Dur, Nitrostat) is a common vasodilator. During vasodilator treatment, you may feel a persistent headache, but it can be relieved with aspirin. Flushing of the neck and head is another common side effect.

- **Thienopyridines.** These drugs include ticlopidine (Ticlid) and clopidogrel (Plavix). They interfere with the production of another substance involved in blood clotting, called adenosine diphosphate. Side effects may include diarrhea, rash, nausea, or vomiting.
- **Glycoprotein IIb/IIIa inhibitors.** This class of drugs includes abciximab (Reopro) and eptifibatide (Integrilin). It prevents clots by interfering with a receptor on the surface of blood platelets, preventing certain proteins from binding to blood platelets and assisting in clotting. These drugs are given intravenously. Side effects may include nausea, vomiting, irritation at the injection site, or dizziness.

Surgery: The most common surgical procedures performed for atherosclerosis are:

- *Angioplasty with stenting.* This procedure is not as invasive as surgery. It is usually performed on an outpatient basis and involves the insertion of a small balloon through a *catheter* into the narrowed blood vessel. The balloon is inflated to open the clogged artery, then a tiny mesh tube called a stent is inserted. The stent remains in the artery to keep it open.
- *Coronary bypass surgery.* During this procedure, the surgeon uses healthy arteries or veins from other areas in your body to bypass the diseased *coronary arteries*.
- *Carotid artery surgery.* In this procedure, the surgeon removes plaque from the carotid artery in the neck to improve blood flow to the brain.

Test Your Knowledge

Answer the following questions to see how much you learned about atherosclerosis.

1. The innermost layer of the artery is called:
   a. Plaque b. Endothelium
   c. Atherosclerotic d. Clots

2. The primary symptoms of atherosclerosis are:
   a. High blood pressure b. High cholesterol
   c. Angina d. Shortness of breath

3. What does an ankle/brachial index measure?
   a. Blood pressure b. Cholesterol
   c. Atherosclerosis d. Blood flow through the body

4. What does a C-reactive protein, or CRP, test measure?
   a. Inflammation b. Blood flow through the body
   c. Cholesterol d. Angina

5. If you have unstable angina, drugs may be prescribed to reduce:
   a. Clotting b. Plaque build up
   c. Headaches d. Shortness of breath

Answers: 1.b 2.c 3.d 4.a 5.a

Hypertension

70 million Americans suffer from high blood pressure.

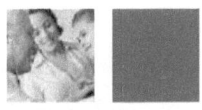
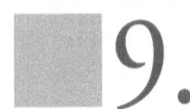

9.

Your blood pressure is the force of blood against your artery walls. When blood pressure stays consistently high for a long time, it is called hypertension.

Causes: There are three major types of *hypertension*:

- Essential hypertension: This is the most common type of high blood pressure, and there is no treatable cause behind it.
- Secondary hypertension: Unlike essential hypertension, this type may be caused by kidney disorders, *congenital* abnormalities, or other medical conditions. Once these conditions are treated, your blood pressure should return to normal levels.
- Pregnancy related hypertension: Some women develop high blood pressure due to pregnancy, called gestational hypertension. In addition, women who already have high blood pressure and who become pregnant may develop more severe hypertension, particularly in the last three months of pregnancy.

Symptoms: Hypertension is called the "silent killer" because it typically has no symptoms. However, some people may feel fatigue, dizziness, or *palpitations*.

Diagnosis: The only way to detect high blood pressure is with regular blood pressure checks. Blood pressure is evaluated with a *sphygmomanometer*, a device that measures your pressure in millimeters of mercury (mm Hg). You've undoubtedly had your pressure measured many times. The inflatable cuff is wrapped around your arm and inflated briefly to squeeze the blood vessels in your arm; when the cuff is released and blood rushes through, the *systolic* and *diastolic* pressure levels are measured. Blood pressure is defined in two numbers: systolic, the first number, which measures the pressure when your heart contracts; and diastolic, which measures the pressure when the heart rests between beats.

- Normal blood pressure is a *systolic pressure* less than 120 mm Hg or a diastolic pressure of 80 mm Hg or less.
- Prehypertension is a systolic pressure of 120 to 139 mm Hg or a diastolic pressure of 80 to 89 mm Hg. Prehypertension means you are at risk of developing hypertension.

- Hypertension is a systolic blood pressure of 140 mm Hg or higher, a diastolic pressure of 90 mm Hg or higher, or both.

Treatment: As with any cardiovascular related condition, lifestyle changes are your first line of defense. Check out Chapter 5 for steps you can take to reduce your blood pressure. I also recommend you purchase a home blood pressure monitor so you can regularly monitor your blood pressure.

You have two options: an aneroid or a digital monitor. An aneroid monitor is more convenient, smaller, and less expensive, costing about $20 to $30. Digital monitors cost up to about $100, but they're easier to use, easier to read, and, thus, more popular. Often, insurance covers the cost of a monitor.

Medications are often a part of hypertension treatment. These include:

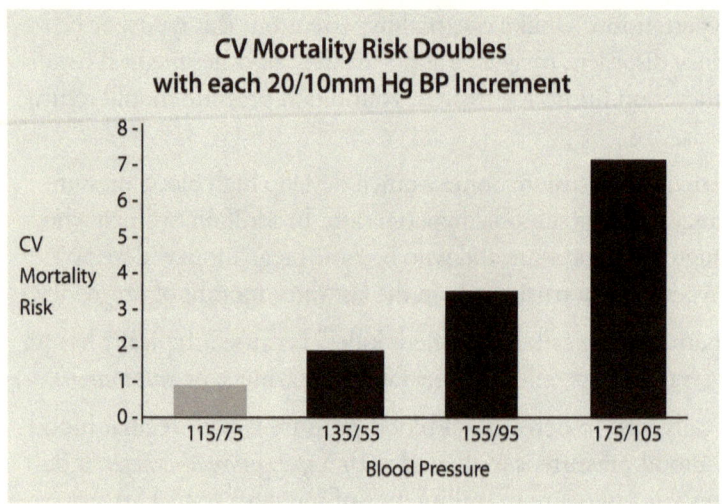

- **Beta-blockers:** Commonly prescribed beta-blockers include atenolol (Tenormin), carvedilol (Coreg), and betaxolol (Kerlone). These drugs reduce nerve impulses to the heart and blood vessels, slowing the heart's beating and reducing its force. Side effects may include diarrhea, abdominal cramps, or nausea.

- **Diuretics:** Commonly prescribed diuretics include triamterene (Dyrenium), furosemide (Lasix), and hydrochlorothiazide (Esidrix). Sometimes called "water pills," these medications work with the kidneys to flush excess sodium and water from your body. Side effects may include dehydration and abnormalities in the blood chemistries, such as potassium loss.

- **Angiotensin–converting enzyme (ACE) inhibitors:** Commonly prescribed ACE inhibitors include captopril (Capoten), benazepril (Lotensin), and enalapril (Vasotec). These medications relax the blood vessels and prevent release of a hormone called *angiotensin II*, which causes blood vessels to narrow. Side effects may include cough, elevated blood potassium levels, low blood pressure, and dizziness.

- **Angiotensin II antagonists:** Valsartan (Diovan) diltiazem (Cardizem), verapamil, amlodipine (Norvasc), nisoldipine (Sular), nifedipine (Adalat, Procardia), and nicardipine (Cardene). By preventing calcium from entering cells in the blood vessels and heart, these medications help blood vessels relax. Side effects may include constipation, low blood pressure, and nausea.

- **Alpha-blockers:** Doxazosin (Cardura) is a commonly prescribed alpha-blocker. This medication relaxes blood vessels and keeps them open, enabling blood to pass through more easily. Side effects may include dizziness, headaches, and tiredness.

- **Alpha-beta-blockers:** This class of drugs includes labetalol (Normodyne, Trandate). Drugs in this class serve the same function as alpha-blockers, but they also help slow the heartbeat, which means less blood is pumped through blood vessels. Side effects may include fatigue, dizziness, and diarrhea.

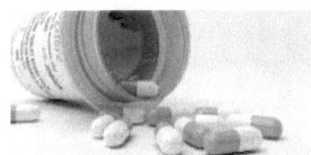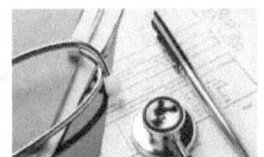

- **Nervous system inhibitors:** This class of drugs includes carvedilol (Coreg). It works by controlling nerve impulses, relaxing and widening blood vessels. Side effects may include dizziness, edema (fluid accumulation), and reduced heart rate.

- **Vasodilators:** The most commonly prescribed vasodilator is nitroglycerin (Nitro-Bid, Nitro-Dur, Nitrostat).

Vasodilators open blood vessels by relaxing vessel walls. Side effects may include persistent headaches and flushing of the neck and head.

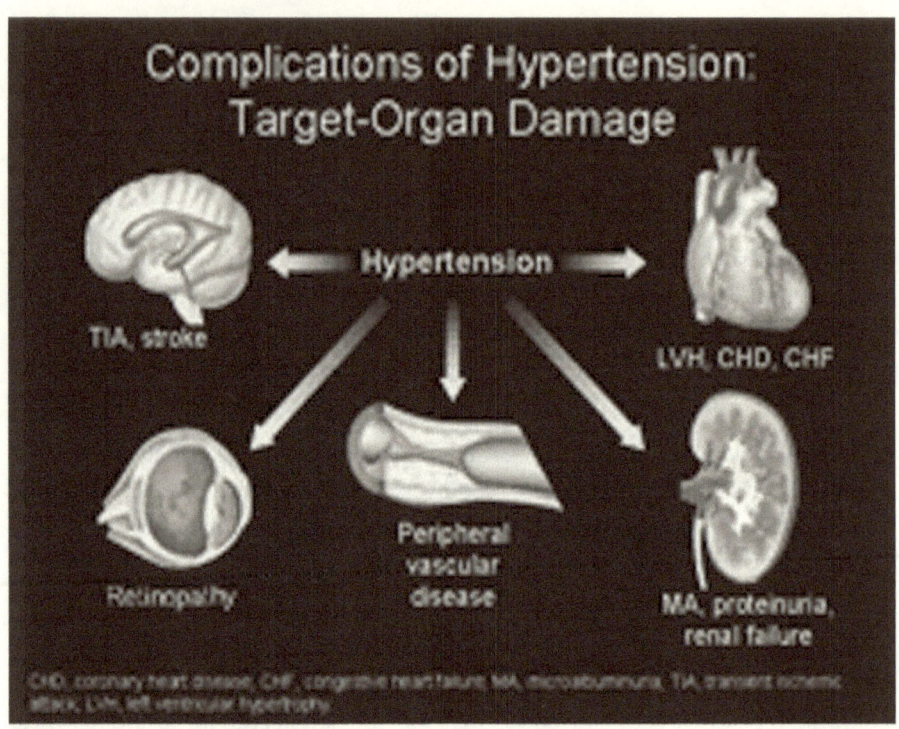

Test Your Knowledge

Answer the following questions to see how much you learned about high blood pressure.

1. We know exactly what causes most cases of hypertension.
   a. True
   b. False

2. Symptoms of hypertension may include:
   a. Headache
   b. Dizziness
   c. Tiredness
   d. All of the above

3. Which drugs reduce nerve impulses to the heart and blood vessels, slowing the heart's beating?
   a. Beta blockers
   b. Alpha blockers
   c. Vasodilators
   d. Ace inhibitors

4. Which drugs prevent the release of a hormone that causes blood vessels to narrow?
   a. Beta blockers
   b. Alpha blockers
   c. Vasodilators
   d. ACE inhibitors

Answers: 1.b 2.d 3.a 4.d

Hyperlipidemia

Keep your bad cholesterol (LDL) under 100!

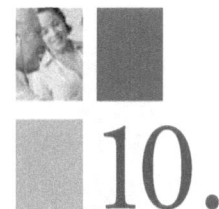

10.

Hyperlipidemia is just the medical term for high lipid levels, commonly referred to as "high *cholesterol.*" *Lipids* are the fats in your blood. Higher than normal levels mean you have higher than normal amounts of cholesterol and *triglycerides* in your blood. (Remember, triglycerides make up most of the fats in your blood; cholesterol is a specific kind of fatty substance. If your triglycerides are high, your total cholesterol usually is, too—and vice versa.)

Cause: Hyperlipidemia is almost always caused by certain medical conditions or lifestyle habits. Lifestyle factors include obesity, lack of physical activity, and smoking. However, diabetes, kidney disease, and an underactive or malfunctioning thyroid are also potential causes.

Heredity presents a risk as well—it's possible to "inherit" high cholesterol from your parents, even if you don't have any of the typical risk factors. Obtaining an accurate family history as described in Chapter 6 is important in determining your risk for high cholesterol.

Age also plays a role. Men over 45 and women over 55 have an increased risk.

Symptoms: High cholesterol doesn't have any symptoms. That's why regular screenings are so important.

Diagnosis: Determining whether you have high cholesterol is as simple as taking a blood test. The National Cholesterol Education Program (NCEP) recommends everyone have their lipid levels tested every five years after age 20.

Ideal results are:
- LDL less than 100 mg/dL
- HDL greater than 40 mg/dL for men and 50 mg/dL for women
- Total cholesterol less than 200 mg/dL
- Triglycerides less than 150 mg/dL

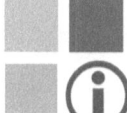

Remember

You fast for 12 hours before the blood test to ensure an accurate measure.

The tables below provide more specifics for your total cholesterol and LDL levels.

Total Cholesterol Level	Category
Less than 200 mg/dL	Desirable
200–239 mg/dL	Borderline high
240 mg/dL and above	High

HDL Cholesterol Level	Category
Less than 40 mg/dL (men)/ less than 50 mg/dL (women)	Low (undesirable)
40–50 mg/dL (men)/ 50–60 mg/dL (women)	Average
60 mg/dL and above	High (desirable)

LDL Cholesterol Level	Category
Less than 100 mg/dL	Optimal
100-129 mg/dL	Near optimal/above optimal
130-159	Borderline high
160-189	High
190 and above	Very high

LDL Cholesterol Level	Category
Less than 150 mg/dL	Normal
150–199 mg/dL	Borderline high
200–499 mg/dL	High
500 mg/dL	Very High

Keep in mind that these numbers are only guidelines. Depending on your medical history, you may need to aim for even lower levels of total and LDL cholesterol and triglycerides to further reduce your risk of coronary disease.

Treatment: If your cholesterol levels are high, lifestyle changes like those described in Chapter 4 are the first step, followed by medications, including:

- **Statins.** Currently, there are five statins on the market: lovastatin (Mevacor), simvastatin (Zocor), pravastatin (Pravachol), rosuvas-tatin (Crestor), and atorvastatin (Lipitor). These drugs slow the production of cholesterol while increasing the liver's ability to remove LDL cholesterol already in the blood. Studies find these drugs can lower LDL cholesterol levels 20 to 60 percent within four to six weeks. Side effects are rare but may include upset stomach, gas, constipation, abdominal pain or cramps, muscle or joint pain, and high liver enzymes.

- **Niacin.** Niacin works in the liver to reduce the production of blood fats. It helps reduce triglyceride and LDL cholesterol levels and increase HDL cholesterol. Stick to prescription niacin—over-the-counter niacin may contain varying amounts. Your options for prescription niacin include Niacor, Niaspan, and Slo-Niacin. Two common side effects include flushing and hot flashes as your blood vessels open more widely than usual. This can be reduced by taking the drug after or during a meal. Other side effects may include itching, nausea, gas, diarrhea, vomiting, or indigestion.

- **Bile acid sequestrants.** These drugs help increase HDL levels as well as reduce LDL levels by binding with cholesterol-containing bile acids in the intestines so they are eliminated when you go to the bathroom. The three most common brands are Questran (cholestyramine), WelChol (colesevelam), and Colestid (colestipol). Bile acid sequestrants come in powder or tablet form—the powder must be mixed with water or fruit juice, and the tablet should be taken with lots of fluids to prevent gastrointestinal issues. However, you may still experience side effects such as gas, nausea, bloating, and constipation.

- **Fibrates.** These drugs help raise HDL levels and lower triglyceride levels by reducing the liver's production of triglyceride-carrying particles called VLDLs and speeding up the removal of triglycerides from the blood. Two of the more common fibrates are Lopid (gemfibrozil) and Tricor (fenofibrate). Side effects may include nausea, upset stomach, and diarrhea.

- **Ezetimibe.** Sold under the brand name Zetia, this drug reduces LDL cholesterol levels by reducing the absorption of cholesterol from the intestine. Side effects are rare, but may include back and joint pain, diarrhea, and sinusitis.

Test Your Knowledge

Take this quiz to see how much you know about high cholesterol.

1. Causes of hyperlipidemia include all of the following except:
    a. High blood pressure
    b. Obesity
    c. Smoking
    d. Diabetes

2. You can "inherit" high cholesterol levels, even if you're otherwise healthy.
    a. True
    b. False

3. You should have your cholesterol levels tested every ____ years after age 20.
    a. 2
    b. 4
    c. 5
    d. 10

4. Lipitor is a(n):
    a. Anticoagulant
    b. Diuretic
    c. Beta blocker
    d. Statin

5. Which cholesterol drug could lead to flushing and hot flashes?
    a. Zocor
    b. Lipitor
    c. Niacin
    d. Questran

Answers: 1.a 2.a 3.c 4.d 5.c

Diabetes and the Heart

Patients with Diabetes are more likely to die of heart disease than from anything else!

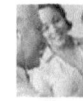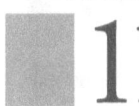

11.

Type 2 diabetes occurs when the cells in your body become resistant to insulin or when specialized cells in your pancreas don't produce enough insulin. Insulin is the hormone required to move glucose produced from food from the bloodstream into cells where it can be used to produce energy. If the glucose can't get into cells, it builds up in your blood, leading to high blood sugar levels. In the meantime, those pancreatic cells keep pumping out more insulin to get that glucose into cells. Not only can the high insulin/ glucose levels damage blood vessels, but the pancreatic cells responsible for making insulin may eventually wear out.

> Insulin acts like a doorman, only instead of allowing guests in the lobby doors, it allows glucose through the cell membrane!

Ninety percent of all diabetes is type 2 diabetes (type 1 occurs when the immune system destroys the insulin-producing cells in the pancreas). If you have type 2 diabetes, you're more likely to die from heart disease than from anything else, and at least twice as likely as someone without diabetes to have heart disease or a stroke. In fact, the link between diabetes and heart disease is so strong that if you have diabetes, you should be treated as if you also have heart disease.

Cause: Type 2 diabetes is associated with age, obesity, family history, physical inactivity and impaired glucose metabolism.

Symptoms: There are often no symptoms for type 2 diabetes, but they can include thirst, weight loss, blurry eyesight, and frequent urination. In many cases, the diagnosis occurs even before the symptoms begin.

Diagnosis: Diabetes is diagnosed with one of the following blood tests:

- **Fasting plasma glucose test.** This is the preferred test for diabetes. Your blood glucose levels are measured after eight hours of fasting. A glucose level of 100 to 125 mg/dL means you are at risk of developing diabetes (pre-diabetes), while a level of 126 mg/dL or above means you have diabetes.

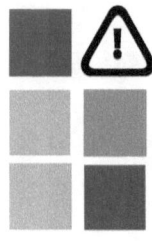

CAUTION! One danger with diabetes is that it can damage the nerves that send pain signals to the brain, so you can have heart disease or even a heart attack without experiencing the typical symptoms of chest pain or pressure, pounding heartbeat, or jaw or arm pain. Thus, it's very important that you schedule regular check-ups to carefully monitor your condition.

- **Oral plasma glucose test.** This test is also conducted after eight hours of fasting. Then you drink a beverage containing 75 grams of glucose. Two hours later, your plasma glucose levels are measured. A blood glucose level between 140 and 199 mg/dL puts you at risk of developing diabetes, while a level of 200 mg/ dL or above indicates diabetes, checks blood glucose after you drink a glucose beverage, but at random times.
- **Random plasma glucose test.** A random plasma glucose test above 200 mg/dL indicates diabetes.

Treatment: All treatments for diabetes focus on helping you manage your blood sugar levels. Levels are measured with a hemoglobin A1C test, a blood test that provides a snapshot of your glucose levels over the past three months. The goal is to maintain an A1C level of seven or lower.

In addition to the lifestyle changes covered in Chapter 5, you may need the following oral medications to help you maintain normal blood sugar levels:

- **Sulfonylureas.** These drugs, including glimepiride (Amyrol), glyburide (Diabeta), and tolazamide, trigger the pancreas to make more insulin. Taking them increases your risk of hypoglycemia, or low blood sugar, with symptoms like nausea, tiredness, hunger, *palpitations*, and headache. Other side effects include heartburn and diarrhea, but those can sometimes be avoided by taking the medication with a meal.
- **Biguanides.** This class of drugs includes glucophage (Metformin). They tell the liver to decrease its production of glucose, which increases glucose levels in the blood. Since it doesn't increase insulin levels, this drug carries little to no risk of hypoglycemia. Also, glucophage can act as an appetite suppressant, so it often helps you lose weight.
- **Alpha-glucosidase inhibitors.** These drugs include acarbose (Precose). They reduce the amount of carbohydrates your digestive tract absorbs,

reducing after-meal glucose levels. Because these drugs work with the digestive system, possible side effects include abdominal pain, diarrhea, and gas.

- **Thiazolidinediones.** This class of drugs includes rosiglitazone (Avandia), pioglitazone (Actos), and troglitazone (Rezulin). They help insulin work better at the cellular level. In essence, they make your cells more sensitive to insulin. The most common side effects include upper respiratory tract infection, headache, back pain, hypoglycemia, and sinusitis. They may also cause weight gain.

- **Meglinitides.** These drugs include repaglinide (Prandin) and nateglinide (Starlix). They trigger the pancreas to make more insulin depending on the blood level of glucose. Potential side effects may include hypoglycemia, flu-like symptoms, nausea, vomiting, or headache.

If you continue to have poor blood glucose control despite lifestyle changes and oral medications, you may need insulin, which is injected under the skin, Insulin preparations differ in how fast they start to work and how long they work. It may take some time to determine the best type to use and the best time to use it. You may also need to mix more than one type in the syringe. Be patient!

We will figure out the best way to control your blood sugar, thus reducing your risk of heart disease.

One Patient's Story

Stephanie Sanchez, 36, has diabetes. After undergoing gallbladder surgery, she returned home and began to feel what she described as "congestion" in her chest. She also experienced shortness of breath. Two days after the gallbladder surgery, she was rushed back to the hospital. There, I found she'd had a massive heart attack during the gallbladder surgery. An angiogram showed all of her heart arteries were blocked, requiring an emergency quadruple bypass surgery. Her heart was damaged so badly she had to be kept in the ICU for more than two months.

Test Your Knowledge

Answer the following questions to see how much you learned about diabetes.

1. Most people with diabetes have type 1 diabetes, in which their insulin-producing cells stop working:
    a. True
    b. False

2. The main cause of death for someone with type 2 diabetes is:
    a. High blood sugar
    b. Kidney failure
    c. Nerve damage
    d. Heart disease or stroke

3. The best test for diagnosing diabetes is the:
    a. Fasting plasma glucose test
    b. Oral plasma glucose test
    c. Random plasma glucose test
    d. Urine glucose test

4. The ideal A1C level in someone with diabetes is:
    a. Less than 5 percent
    b. Less than 7 percent
    c. Less than 9 percent
    d. Less than 10 percent

5. Which drug or type of drug helps your pancreas make more insulin?
    a. Metformin
    b. Sulfonylureas
    c. Injectable insulin
    d. Precose

Answers: 1.b 2.d 3.a 4.b 5.b

Peripheral Artery Disease

Do you have difficulty walking?

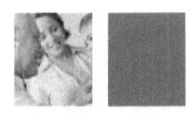
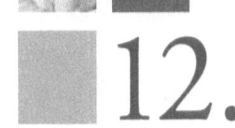

12.

Definition: *Peripheral artery disease*, also known as PAD or leg artery disease, is a condition in which the arteries in your legs become blocked with plaque, preventing your legs and feet from receiving enough blood.

Symptoms: Most people with PAD experience *intermittent claudication* (IC). This is discomfort or pain in your legs when you walk or move that disappears when you stay off your feet. Intermittent claudication may not always feel painful. Sometimes, it might feel like a tightness, heaviness, cramping, or weakness in your leg.

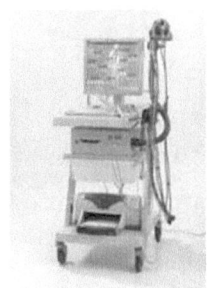

If you have advanced PAD, you may experience *critical limb ischemia*, which occurs when your legs don't get enough oxygen even when you're at rest, leading to pain in your feet or toes. In the most severe cases of PAD, you develop painful sores on your toes or feet from lack of oxygenated blood. If the circulation in your legs doesn't improve, these ulcers could lead to gangrene, and you could lose your toes, foot, or even your leg.

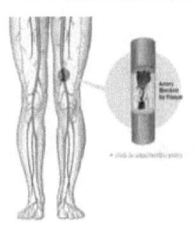

Definition: *Peripheral artery disease*, also known as PAD or leg artery disease, is a condition in which the arteries in your legs become blocked with plaque, preventing your legs and feet from receiving enough blood.

Symptoms: Most people with PAD experience *intermittent claudication* (IC). This is discomfort or pain in your legs when you walk or move that disappears when you stay off your feet. Intermittent claudication may not always feel painful. Sometimes, it might feel like a tightness, heaviness, cramping, or weakness in your leg.

If you have advanced PAD, you may experience *critical limb ischemia*, which occurs when your legs don't get enough oxygen even when you're at rest, leading to pain in your feet or toes. In the most severe cases of PAD, you develop painful sores on your toes or feet from lack of oxygenated blood. If the circulation in your legs doesn't improve, these ulcers could lead to gangrene, and you could lose your toes, foot, or even your leg.

Causes: The main cause of peripheral artery disease is atherosclerosis. Just as your risk of developing atherosclerosis increases as you get older, so does your risk of PAD. If you're over 50 or are male, you have a higher risk than younger people or women.

Other risk factors include smoking, diabetes, high blood pressure, high cholesterol, high triglycerides, and high levels of homocysteine, an amino acid that indicates *inflammation*. If you weigh 30 percent or more than your ideal weight or your body mass index (BMI) is 28 or higher, you also have an increased risk for PAD. (See BMI charts on page 45.)

Diagnosis: Tests for PAD include:

- *Ankle/brachial index.* This simple test measures the blood pressure in your ankles and right arm—the brachial artery. It compares the mean systolic blood pressure in each ankle to the mean *systolic pressure* in your arm. Your ankle pressure should be at least 90 percent of your arm pressure. A pressure less than 50 percent indicates severe narrowing of the arteries in your legs.

- **Cholesterol test.** You fast for 12 hours before this simple blood test, which measures cholesterol and other blood fat levels in your blood.

- **Duplex ultrasound.** This noninvasive test uses sound waves to visualize the artery while measuring the blood flow to the artery. It helps detect any abnormalities or blockages in blood vessels.

- **Pulse-volume recording.** This test uses an arm pressure cuff and a Doppler probe, a tool that transmits sound waves into your body and creates a tracing of your blood vessels, to measure the volume of blood in your legs.

- **Magnetic resonance angiography (MRA).** This test uses magnetic fields and radio waves to depict blockages in your arteries.

- **Angiography.** In an *angiography*, a catheter is inserted through your groin or arm and a contrast dye injected through it into your bloodstream to highlight the arteries. This procedure is used only for people with the most severe forms of PAD. It takes about 30 minutes, but you'll be monitored for about four hours afterward to make sure you're OK. (You'll find more information about this test in Chapter 5.)

Treatment: As with all cardiovascular-related conditions, lifestyle changes are critical. One that might sound counter intuitive is exercise. But walking short distances three to four times a week, with intervals of rest built in, can make a tremendous difference.

Dr. Kumar recommends starting such a program through a rehabilitation center, but if that isn't possible, we'll work with you to develop a program you can follow.

Medication: Specific medications prescribed for PAD include:

- **Antiplatelet medications.** These include aspirin and clopidogrel (Plavix). They work by making your blood platelets less likely to stick to each other and form blood clots. Possible side effects include stomach ulcers, abdominal pain, nausea, and *gastritis*.
- **Anticoagulant medications.** These drugs, which include heparin and warfarin (Coumadin), also prevent blood clots. They work by inactivating clotting factors in your blood, as well as by preventing your liver from producing chemicals required for clotting.
- **Statins.** These cholesterol-lowering medications can slow the progression of PAD while also improving claudication symptoms. Lovastatin (Mecavor), simvastatin (Zocor), pravastatin (Pravachol), rosuvastatin (Crestor), and atorvastatin (Lipitor) are all options. Statins work by inhibiting an enzyme in the liver necessary for cholesterol production. Possible side effects include headache, nausea, vomiting, constipation, and diarrhea.
- **Cilostazol (Pletal).** This medication helps increase physical activity by reducing the pain of claudication. It dilates the arteries and increases the supply of oxygenated blood to the arms and legs. Side effects are mild, including headache, diarrhea, or dizziness.
- **Pentoxifylline (Pentoxil, Trental).** This drug improves blood and oxygen delivery to vital tissues. Possible side effects include nausea, headaches, anxiety, loss of appetite, and insomnia.

One Patient's Story

Cindy, 40, came to see me because she was experiencing pains in her legs. "It was horrible," she said. "Trying to walk the mall at Christmas ... forget it. I just couldn't do it." I evaluated her, finding she had a significantly blocked artery in her leg. He performed angioplasty to open the artery using a special catheter that "shaves" the plaque from the blood vessel. She was home that evening and is now walking without pain. The plaque collects in the tip of the catheter and then is completely removed from the body. "It worked," Cindy says of the procedure. "I can walk all the way around the block without stopping."

Procedures: More severe cases of PAD may require surgery or other cardiovascular procedures, including:

- **Bypass surgery.** In this surgical procedure, the surgeon uses a healthier artery from your leg to create an alternate route around a narrowed or blocked section of a leg artery.
- **Endarterectomy.** In this procedure, the surgeon removes plaque from your leg arteries to improve blood flow and circulation.
- *Angioplasty with stenting.* This procedure is not as invasive as surgery. It is usually performed on an outpatient basis and involves inserting a small balloon through a catheter into the narrowed blood vessel. The balloon is inflated to open the clogged artery, then a tiny mesh tube called a *stent* is inserted. The stent remains in the artery to keep it open.

Test Your Knowledge

Answer the following questions to see how much you have learned about peripheral artery disease.

1. Angioplasty often involves:
   a. Major surgery   b. General anesthesia
   c. A stent   d. Open-heart surgery

2. In which procedure does the surgeon remove plaque from your leg artery?
   a. Angioplasty   b. Bypass surgery
   c. Endarterectomy   d. Colonoscopy

3. Which drug is not designed to prevent blood clots?
   a. Statins   b. Aspirin
   c. Plavix   d. Heparin

4. Which test involves the use of dye?
   a. Ultrasound   b. Angiography
   c. X-ray   d. Pulse-volume recording

5. Which test measures the blood pressure in your leg?
   a. Pulse-volume recording   b. MRA
   c. Ankle/brachial index   d. Blood pressure tests:

Answers:
1. c 2. c 3. a 4. b 5. c

Congestive Heart Failure

Is your heart pumping enough blood?

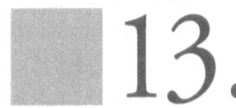

13.

Definition: *Congestive heart failure* means your heart doesn't pump enough blood to keep your body working as it should. It sounds scary, and rightly so. According to the American Heart Association, nearly 5 million Americans are living with heart failure, and 550,000 new cases are diagnosed each year.

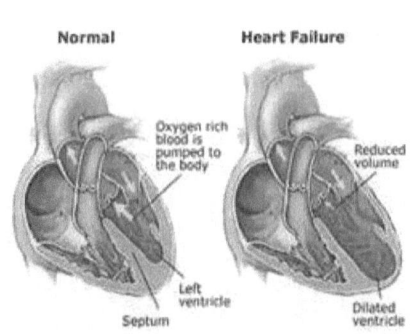

If you have this condition, your heart beats faster than normal to try and make up for the missing blood. The *ventricles*, which are the heart chambers that receive blood, then push the blood into arteries in the heart, which stretch to accommodate more blood. As a result, you have difficulty exerting yourself physically because you tire more easily and experience shortness of breath because you're not getting enough oxygenated blood.

Cause: Heart failure is a chronic condition that typically occurs after other conditions have weakened the heart. Heart failure can affect the right, left, or both sides of the heart.

Causes include smoking, poor diet, alcohol, high blood pressure, *cholesterol*, and diabetes. In addition, physical changes to the heart also increase your risk. For instance, if you've suffered a *heart attack* or have structural cardiac defects such as abnormal valves, you have a higher risk of heart failure.

Sometimes, however, your heart weakens without a specific cause. This is called *idiopathic dilated cardiomyopathy*.

In congestive heart failure, the heart doesn't pump blood as it should, so the blood often pools in areas below the heart, including the liver, legs, feet, ankles, gastrointestinal tract, arms, and legs (known as *right-sided heart failure*), or in the lungs (known as *left-sided heart failure*).

Your kidneys might also retain excess water and sodium. Left-sided failure can cause right-sided failure as extra pressure in the lungs is eventually passed to the right side of the heart, which then fails.

Heart failure may also be *systolic* (when the *left ventricle* does not contract or pump blood properly), *diastolic* (when the left ventricle loses its ability to relax or fill fully), or a combination of both. Diagnosing the correct type of heart failure is important since it determines the type of treatment and medication you need.

Symptoms:

- Fatigue
- Weakness
- Shortness of breath during activities and while lying down
- Coughing and wheezing
- Swelling in the legs, ankles, feet, or abdomen
- Sudden weight gain
- Lack of appetite and/or nausea
- Inability to exercise
- Lack of concentration

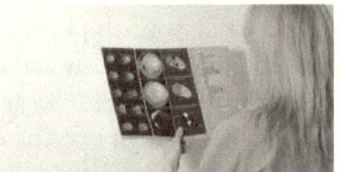

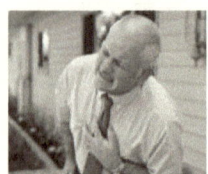

Diagnosis: The first steps in diagnosing congestive heart failure are a physical exam, blood test, and chest X-ray. The blood test identifies heart diseases and evaluates liver and thyroid functions. High levels of the hormone *brain natriuretic peptide* (BNP) may indicate that you have heart failure.

Other tests include many of those discussed in previous chapters, such as an *echocardiogram*, *electrocardiogram* (ECG), and coronary catheterization (*angiogram*). Some tests, including *radionuclide ventriculography or multiple gated acquisition scan* (MUGA), involve injecting radioactive material into your blood to help identify problems. Each shows how well the heart chambers work, as well as how much blood is in the heart. The tests also measure your *ejection fraction*, which shows how much blood your heart pumps out. If the chambers don't pump enough blood, you may have heart failure.

If you've been diagnosed with mild or moderate heart failure, you need to see Dr. Kumar or other cardiologists every three to six months for cardiac evaluation. You also need to monitor your condition at home with daily weigh-ins. If you're gaining more than 5 pounds in a week it can be your condition is worsening.

Treatment: Medications are the most common treatment for heart failure. They include:

- **ACE inhibitors.** These include captopril (Capoten) and enalapril (Vasotec). They work by opening blood vessels, thus relieving pressure on the heart. Side effects include a persistent dry cough, abdominal pain, diarrhea, fatigue, and dizziness.
- **Diuretics.** These include thiazide, loop diuretics, and potassium-sparing diuretics. They work by reducing the amount of fluid and sodium in your blood, which reduces pressure on your heart. When you start taking a diuretic, you may experience some dizziness. Other side effects include loss of appetite, headache, or blurred vision.
- **Digitalis.** This drug improves the heart's ability to contract and prevents irregular heart rhythms. Side effects include nausea, diarrhea, loss of appetite, and drowsiness.
- **Angiotensin receptor blockers (ARBs).** These drugs include losartan (Cozaar) and valsartan (Diovan). They prevent the enzyme *angiotensin II* from compressing arteries and veins, which increases blood pressure. These medications are typically prescribed if you're unable to take ACE inhibitors. Side effects include muscle cramps, dizziness, and diarrhea.
- **Beta-blockers.** These drugs include atenolol (Tenormin) and bisoprolol (Zebeta). They work by slowing your heart rate and reducing blood pressure. They also help reduce irregular heart rhythms, improving overall heart function. Side effects include abdominal cramps, diarrhea, and dizziness.

To help manage congestive heart failure, it's important that you:

- Take all medications regularly and as prescribed
- Limit salt and sodium intake.
- Quit smoking.
- Exercise and maintain a healthy weight.

Test Your Knowledge

Answer the following questions to see how much you have learned about heart failure.

1. Suddenly gaining weight is a danger sign if you have congestive heart failure because:
   a. It means you are eating too much.
   b. It means you are eating too much salt.
   c. It means you are retaining fluid.
   d. It means you might get diabetes.

2. Which class of drugs slows your heart rate?
   a. Beta-blockers
   b. ARBs
   c. ACE inhibitors
   d. Digitalis

3. Which drug helps prevent irregular heart rhythms and helps your heart contract better?
   a. Digitalis
   b. Aspirin
   c. Coumadin
   d. Thiazide

4. Which drugs help reduce the amount of fluid and sodium in your blood?
   a. ACE inhibitors
   b. Digitalis
   c. Statins
   d. Diuretics

5. Which of the following measures how much blood your heart pumps out?
   a. Ejection fraction
   b. Cholesterol test
   c. Blood pressure test
   d. Electrocardiogram

Answers:
1. c 2. a 3. a 4. d 5. a

Atrial Fibrillation

Rhythm of your heart matters.

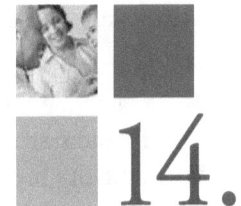

14.

Definition: *Atrial fibrillation* is a form of *arrhythmia*, or a heart rhythm disorder. This condition is associated with a rapid heart rate, in which the heart's upper two chambers (atria) contract abnormally and out of synch with the two lower chambers (ventricles). More than 2 million Americans have atrial fibrillation, which can cause palpitations, shortness of breath, fatigue, and stroke.

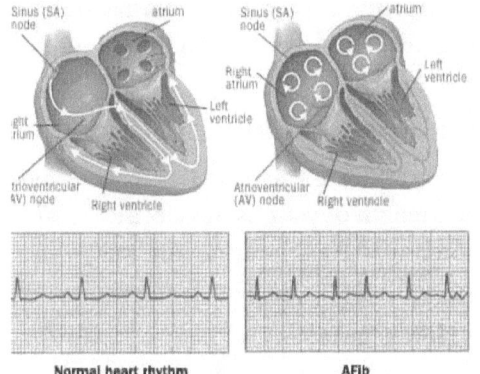

Atrial fibrillation occurs when the heart's electrical signal begins in a different part of the atrium than the sinoatrial node (sinus node) or when the signal is conducted abnormally. Normally the sinus node, which is the heart's pacemaker and regulates contraction, produces an impulse that travels to the atria and then to the atrioventricular node—a path between the upper and lower chambers. The signal causes the atria to contract and then immediately causes the ventricles to contract to pump blood from the heart to the rest of your body.

If the sinus node signal begins improperly, it doesn't travel to the heart in regulated pulses. Instead, it can spread to the atria rapidly and chaotically. This disorganized signal causes the wall of the atrial to fibrillate, or pulsate rapidly. This leads to an abnormally fast heart rate of between 100 to 175 beats per minute, compared to the normal rate of 60 to 100 beats a minute. This faster heart beat prevents proper blood flow to the ventricles and the rest of your body.

Cause: Like all heart diseases, several factors increase your risk for atrial fibrillation, including age, high blood pressure, previous heart attack, abnormal heart valves, congenital heart defects, high blood pressure, smoking, and high alcohol and caffeine intake (think about how your heart speeds up when you drink coffee). *Hyperthyroidism*, in which your thyroid gland produces too much thyroid hormone, also increases your risk.

Symptoms: Atrial fibrillation may start and stop suddenly. They include:

- heart palpitations, in which you can feel your heart beating in your chest
- a racing, pounding, slow, or irregular pulse
- dizziness or fainting
- difficulty breathing and shortness of breath
- fatigue
- a feeling of tightness or squeezing sensation in the chest

Atrial fibrillation can be chronic or sporadic. Sporadic conditions, also called paroxysmal atrial fibrillation, occur if your symptoms are inconsistent. Chronic atrial fibrillation occurs if your symptoms persist until treated.

Diagnosis: The first step in diagnosing atrial fibrillation is conducting a complete physical examination, including measuring your pulse. A normal pulse rate is between 60 and 100 beats per minute. People with atrial fibrillation may have pulse rates between 100 and 175.

Diagnosis: Certain tests may also help detect atrial fibrillation, including:

- **Electrocardiogram.** An electrocardiogram, or EKG, measures the rate and regularity of your heartbeat and the strength of your heart's electric signal. During the test, 12 patches are placed on your chest, arms, and legs. You lie still while the electrodes measure your heart's signal.

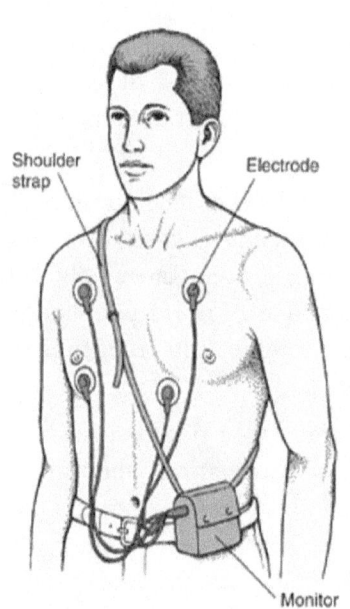

- **Holter monitor.** A Holter monitor is a recorder you wear for an extended time to record your heart's electrical activity. It is also called an ambulatory electrocardiography. Another option is to wear an event recorder. This device is very similar to the Holter monitor except you use a phone to transmit signals to a recorder only when you experience symptoms.

- **Echocardiogram:** This test uses sound waves to create a picture of the blood flow through your heart. After an EKG, a gel is smoothed across your chest and a transducer, which produces high-frequency sound, is placed on your ribs toward the heart. The device "listens" to echoes of the sound emitted from your heart, changing those echoes to electrical impulses to create an image.

- **Stress test:** A stress test is an EKG conducted while you exercise.
- **Angiography:** In a coronary angiography, dye is injected through a catheter into a heart vessel. The dye appears on the X-ray, clearly showing how blood moves through your heart.

Treatment: Atrial fibrillation is typically treated by "resetting" the heart's rhythm. This is done with electrical cardioversion or intravenous drugs.

- **Electrical cardioversion.** This procedure occurs under anesthesia. An electric shock is delivered through paddles placed on your chest to stop your heart's electrical activity for less than a second. Your heart resumes beating, hopefully with a normal rhythm. It's kind of like rebooting a computer.
- **Antiarrhythmic medications.** These drugs include dofetilide (Tikosyn), amiodarone (Cordarone), and ibutilide (Corvert). They are designed to reset your heart's rhythm.
- **Rate-controlling medications.** If antiarrhythmic drugs don't work, you may need beta blockers. These include atenolol (Tenormin), metoprolol (Lopressor, Toprol XL), and propranolol (Inderal). Another alternative is calcium channel blockers, such as diltiazem (Cardizem, Dilacor), amlodipine (Norvasc), or bepridil (Vascor), which are designed to slow the heartbeat.
- **Radiofrequency ablation/pacemaker.** This procedure is performed under sedation on an outpatient basis. Radio frequency energy is used to scar the heart tissue responsible for the abnormal impulse. Sometimes the energy is directed to the atrioventricular junction (the part of the heart that regulates impulses coming from the atria before the ventricles), and a permanent pacemaker is then implanted.

Of course, an atrial pacemaker can also be implanted under the skin to regulate the heart rhythm without the need for radio frequency ablation.

Test Your Knowledge

Answer the following questions to see how much you have learned about atrial fibrillation. Then turn to the next page for the correct answers.

1. The best way to treat atrial fibrillation is:
    a. With statins
    b. With exercise
    c. By resetting the heart's rhythm
    d. With surgery:

2. Delivering an electrical shock to the heart is called:
    a. Electrical cardioversion
    b. Electrical therapy
    c. Echocardiogram
    d. EKG

3. A normal pulse rate is between:
    a. 30 and 60
    b. 60 and 100
    c. 100 and 175
    d. 120 and 150

4. If you can feel your heart beating in your chest, you are having:
    a. A heart attack
    b. A stroke
    c. Angina
    d. Heart palpitations

5. If your heart is fibrillating it is:
    a. Contracting
    b. Beating abnormally rapidly
    c. Beating too slowly
    d. Expanding

Answers:
1. c 2. a 3. b 4. d 5. a

Graphics

Examples of posters and graphics displayed at The Heart Center.

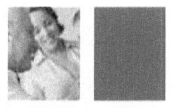

15.

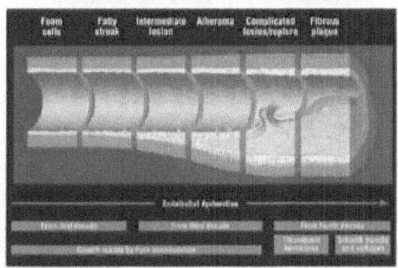

What Causes Heart Attack

Atherosclerosis Timeline

Progression of an Occluding Thrombus

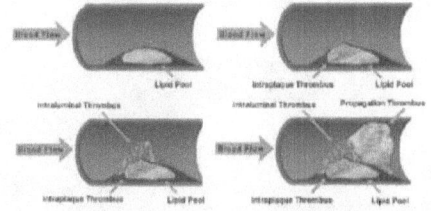

Factoid 1:

Most heart attacks occur because of a blood clot building on top of a ruptured plaque.

Can Heart Attacks Occur at Early Ages of 30's and 40's?

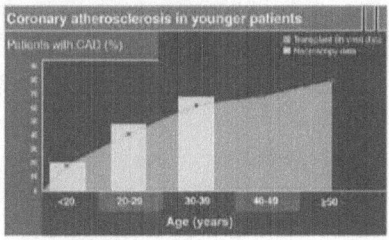

Factoid 2:

Necroscopy data shows affirmation of plaque build up starts early in life and to our surprise up to 70% of people will have plaque by age 40.

 The Heart Center
525 34th Street • Bakersfield, CA 93301

Coronary Artery Disease (CAD)

The Diagnosis Often Comes Too Late.

In almost half of patients, heart attack or death is the initial presentation. A fourth to one half of patients with heart attacks never have any symptoms.

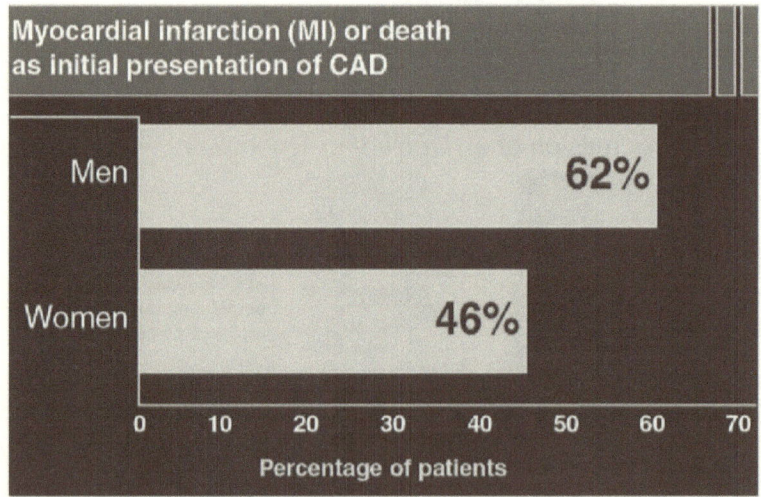

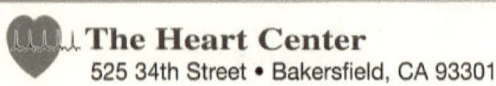

The Heart Center
525 34th Street • Bakersfield, CA 93301

Woman with Heart Disease
47 year old woman with indigestion.

This 55-year old female has been an established patient since June of "96." She came to The Heart Center with symptoms of shortness of breath and chest discomfort. A nuclear scan picked up the problem. Dr. Kumar found 99% blockage in the main artery and opened it with a stent/angioplasty. The procedure was successful and a follow-up nuclear scan showed better perfusion. Patient continues to do well.

Sandra feels grateful for all that Dr. Kumar has done for her and that "if it wasn't for Dr. Kumar, I wouldn't be here today."

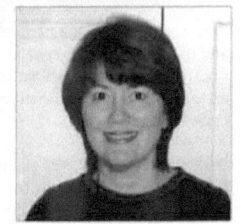

Ms. Sandra Rehkoff

Nuclear Scan BEFORE Angioplasty/Stent

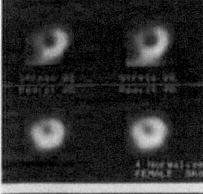

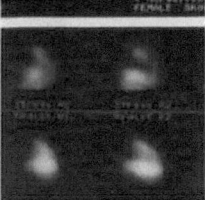

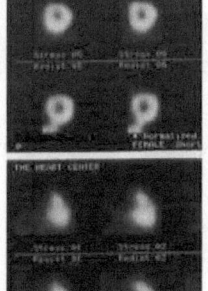

AFTER Angioplasty/Stent

Angioplasty/Stent

BEFORE

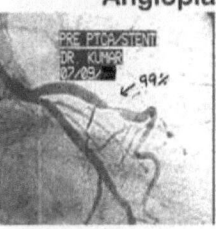

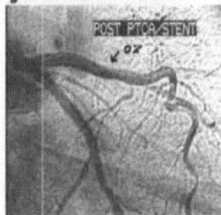

AFTER

 The Heart Center
525 34th Street • Bakersfield, CA 93301

A 58 Year Old Patient with Indigestion and Gas in Chest

Bart came to The Heart Center in 1999 with symptoms of indigestion and gas in the chest. Had a stress test that was normal, then a nuclear scan revealed the problem. Angioplasty revealed 99% blockage in the main artery. Dr. Kumar performed stent/angioplasty and the patient continues to do well.

Bart said he was "very pleased to see how concerned and attentive Dr. Kumar was. That not too many doctors take the time and effort to listen." Bart was very impressed on how little time it took from the initial visit to diagnose that an angiogram procedure was needed. Within days the patient was without any symptoms whatsoever and was back on his way to good health. Bart says that "Dr. Vinod Kumar is a brilliant and caring person and I thank him for saving my life."

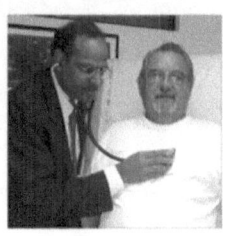

Mr. Bart Estrada

Nuclear Scan

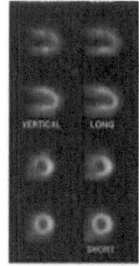

Before / After

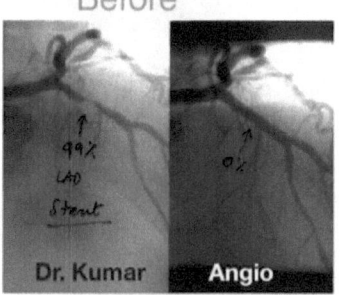

"Heart Attack frequently presents with indigestion and the condition is frequently misdiagnosed as stomach upset, as it did with President Eisenhower in 1955."

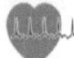

The Heart Center
525 34th Street • Bakersfield, CA 93301

Can you have a Normal Stress Test even with Blocked Arteries?

52 year old man presented with chest congestion. Patient did not improve with antibiotics. Stress test was normal, but the nuclear scan showed abnormalities. Patient had 99.9% blockage in the "widow maker" artery. Dr. Kumar performed Stent/angioplasty in 1999. Patient continues to do well.

Nuclear Scan

Before 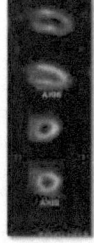 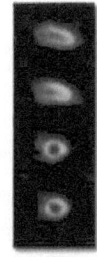 After

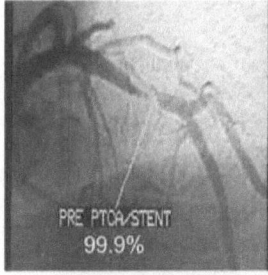 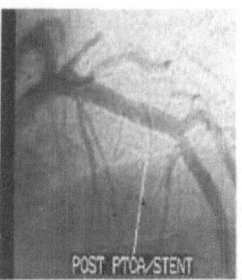

Note: As happened to President Clinton, 1 out of 3 patients with blocked arteries have false negative results on simple stress tests.

 The Heart Center
525 34th Street • Bakersfield, CA 93301

Heart Attack

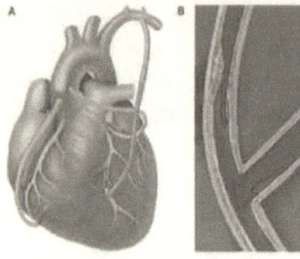

The Heart is a bag of muscles whose main function is to pump. The energy/oxygen to the heart is supplied by 3 major arteries. If there is narrowing in one or more arteries, the heart muscle complains in form of chest pain known as angina. If the artery blocks totally, then it causes damage to heart muscle known as heart attack. A heart attack weakens the heart muscle. This weak pump weakens the body for rest of our life.

56 Year Old White Male with Acute MI

Patient presented with indigestion to San Joaquin Hospital. Patient had an abnormal EKG and was found to have had a heart attack. The patient had 100% blockage and stent/angioplasty saved his life.

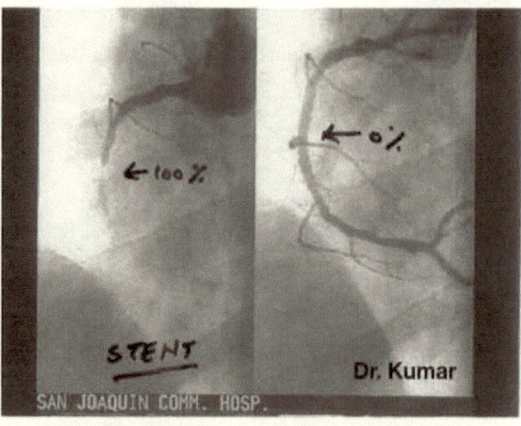

Factoid

In the 1950's, if a patient came into the hospital having suffered a heart attack, chances were only 30% that he would survive. In 2004, the chances are more than 90% that the patient will walk out alive.

 The Heart Center
525 34th Street • Bakersfield, CA 93301

Young People and Heart Disease

35 year old White Male with Chest Pain

He passed the simple stress test twice. However, a nuclear scan here at The Heart Center picked up blockage and patient required 4 vessel coronary bypass surgery.

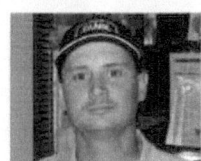

Mr. Bobby Coker

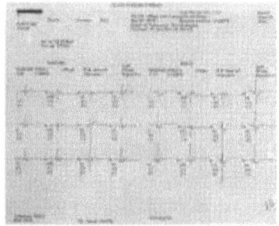

Non-significant Stress Test

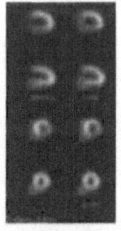

Abnormal Nuclear Scan

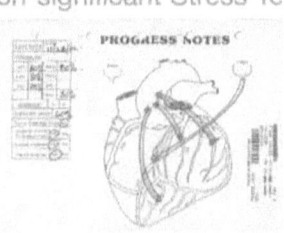

4 Vessel By-pass

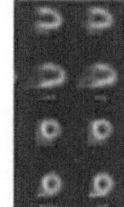

Improved Scan After Surgery

Note: Up to 50% of patients with diabetes have no symptoms of blocked arteries in the heart.

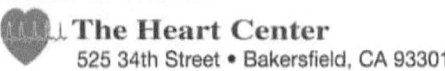

The Heart Center
525 34th Street • Bakersfield, CA 93301

Glossary

Here are their definitions:

adenosine diphosphate: Substance involved in blood clotting.

ambulatory electrocardiography: Records your heart's electrical activity while you do your normal daily activities; see "Holter monitor."

aneurysm: Blood clot in the brain.

angina: Recurring chest pain due to a lack of blood supply to the heart.

angiogram: Procedure in which dye is injected into your bloodstream and observed moving through your blood vessels.

angiography: A procedure used to check for blocked arteries in which an IV is inserted in your arm or groin and a catheter threaded through the IV into the coronary artery. A dye is then injected through the IV/catheter (a "coronary cath") to help the arteries and other heart vessels appear on an X-ray.

angioplasty: Procedure in which a catheter is inserted through your groin into your coronary arteries to clear out plaque.

angioplasty with stenting: Procedure involves inserting a small balloon through a catheter into the narrowed blood vessel. The balloon is inflated to open the clogged artery, then a tiny mesh tube called a stent is inserted. The stent remains in the artery to keep it open.

angiotensin II: An enzyme that causes blood vessels to narrow.

ankle/brachial index: A test to measure the blood pressure in your brachial artery (in your arm) and compare it to the blood pressure in your ankles to show if blood flow is consistent throughout your body.

aorta: The large artery that carries blood from the left ventricle of the heart.

arrhythmia: Abnormal heart beat.

arteriosclerosis: Condition in which the arteries thicken and harden with plaque buildup.

atherosclerosis: Buildup of plaque on artery walls; a form of arteriosclerosis.

atrial fibrillation: A form of arrhythmia, or a heart rhythm disorder. This condition is associated with a rapid heart rate, in which the heart's upper two chambers (atria) contract abnormally and out of synch with the two lower chambers (ventricles).

| 115

atrioventricular junction: The part of the heart that regulates impulses coming from the atria before the ventricles.

atrium: Upper chamber of the heart; there is a right atrium and a left atrium.

autoimmune disease: Diseases that result when the immune system attacks "self" cells as if they were foreign bodies.

body mass index (BMI): A figure that tells you whether your weight is in a healthy range based on your height.

brain natriuretic peptide (BNP): The level of this hormone gets high if you have heart failure.

bruit: An abnormal "whooshing" sound in the heart.

calcium channel blockers: Drugs that prevent calcium from entering heart cells and blood vessel walls.

capillaries: Small blood vessels that carry oxygen and nutrients to your body's cells.

cardiac catheterization: Procedure to check for blocked arteries or measure blood pressure within the heart and the amount of oxygen in your blood. A catheter is inserted through a blood vessel in your arm, groin (upper thigh), or neck and threaded through to your heart. Then an instrument with a camera on the end is snaked through the catheter to show the condition of the arteries.

cardiovascular disease: Conditions affecting the heart and blood vessels.

carotid artery surgery: Procedure in which the surgeon removes plaque from the carotid artery in the neck to improve blood flow to the brain.

catheter: A thin, flexible tube.

chronic atrial fibrillation: Inconsistent atrial fibrillation, or abnormal heart rhythm, that doesn't go away until treated.

cholesterol: Blood fat that can accumulate on artery walls.

computed tomography (CT) scan: A three-dimensional X-ray.

congenital: Born with.

congestive heart failure: Condition in which the heart cannot pump enough blood to the rest of the body.

coronary angiography: Test to observe how blood flows through your heart; performed in conjunction with a cardiac catheterization. In this test, a dye is then injected through the IV/catheter (a "coronary cath") to help the arteries and other heart vessels appear on an X-ray.

coronary arteries: Blood vessels that bring blood and oxygen to the heart.

coronary artery disease: Condition that occurs when the blood vessels that supply blood and oxygen to the heart become narrowed or blocked.

coronary bypass surgery: Surgery in which the surgeon uses healthy arteries or veins from other areas in your body to bypass the diseased coronary arteries.

C-reactive protein (CRP): A blood test that measures a blood protein that shows the presence of inflammation.

critical limb ischemia: Occurs when your legs don't get enough oxygen even when you're at rest, leading to pain in your feet or toes.

CT angiogram: A minimally invasive test that provides a three-dimensional image of your heart and blood vessels. A dye may be inserted through an IV so the scanner can take pictures as the dye moves through your bloodstream to identify blockages or other problems with your coronary arteries or other blood vessels.

diastolic heart failure: When the left ventricle loses its ability to relax or fill fully.

diastolic pressure: Measures blood pressure when your heart relaxes between beats, allowing blood in; it is the lower number in blood pressure measurements.

echocardiogram: A test in which sound waves are used to depict the flow of blood through your heart.

ejection fraction: The amount of blood pumped out of the left ventricle with each heartbeat.

electrical cardioversion: An electric shock is delivered through paddles placed on your chest to stop your heart's electrical activity for less than a second. When the heart restarts, it usually resumes a normal rhythm.

electrocardiogram: Test to measure the heart's rhythm.

endarterectomy: A surgical procedure in which plaque is "shaved" from the leg arteries to improve blood flow and circulation.

endothelium: The innermost layer of the artery.

fibrillate: To pulsate rapidly.

gastritis: Irritation of the stomach or intestines.

heart attack: Plaque lining the arteries bursts open, and blood cells called platelets rush in to repair the spot where the plaque ruptured. This creates blood clots that can block blood flow. If the area of the heart around the blocked artery doesn't receive enough oxygen-rich blood, it dies.

high-density lipoproteins (HDL): "Good" cholesterol that helps rid the body of LDL cholesterol.

Holter monitor: A recorder worn for an extended time to record your heart rhythm as you do your normal activities; used in ambulatory electrocardiography.

homocysteine: A blood marker for inflammation.

hypercholesterolemia: Abnormal cholesterol levels.

hyperlipidemia: High lipid levels, commonly called "high cholesterol"; lipids are the fats in your blood.

hypertension: High blood pressure.

hyperthyroidism: Condition in which your thyroid gland produces too much thyroid hormone.

idiopathic dilated cardiomyopathy: When your heart weakens without a specific cause.

inflammation: Results when the immune system rushes in to repair injuries or fight invaders.

intermittent claudication (IC): Discomfort or pain in your legs when you walk or move that disappears when you stay off your feet.

ischemia: Restriction in blood flow to parts of the heart.

left atrium: The part of the heart that collects oxygen-rich blood from the pulmonary veins and contracts to push it into the left ventricle.

left-sided heart failure: In congestive heart failure, when the heart doesn't pump blood as it should and blood pools in the lungs.

left ventricle: The part of the heart that contracts to push oxygen-rich blood out of the heart into the aorta and from there to the rest of the body.

lipids: Fats in your blood.

low-density lipoproteins (LDL): So called "bad" cholesterol that can stick to artery walls.

magnetic resonance imaging (MRI): A diagnostic test that uses magnets to create a three-dimensional picture.

meditation: A stress-reducing exercise in which you sit quietly and try to focus your mind on the moment.

mitochondria: Power plants within cells that produce energy.

mitral valve prolapse: When the valve between the left atrium and left ventricle doesn't open and close properly.

monounsaturated fat: A healthy form of fat found in olive oil and other foods.

multiple gated acquisition scan (MUGA): A procedure that involves injecting radioactive material into the bloodstream to show how well the heart chambers work and how much blood is in the heart and to measure the ejection fraction; also known as radionuclide ventriculography.

myocardial infarction (MI): Heart attack.

myocardium: The heart muscle.

nuclear heart scan: A procedure in which a radioactive material is injected through a vein into the blood stream. As it travels to your heart, special cameras take pictures of it, tracing the blood flow and identifying any blockages.

omega-3 fatty acids: A healthy type of fat found in fish, nuts, and seeds.

pacemaker: A small computerized battery that gives electrical stimulus to the heart to keep it beating when the heart tends to slow or stop.

palpitations: When you can feel your heart beating in your chest.

paroxysmal atrial fibrillation: Inconsistent atrial fibrillation, or abnormal heart rhythm.

peripheral artery disease (PAD): Condition in which the arteries in your legs become blocked with plaque, preventing your legs and feet from receiving enough blood; also known as leg artery disease.

plant sterol esters: Cholesterol like chemicals in plants that can reduce cholesterol levels in humans.

plaque: Cholesterol, calcium, and cellular debris that builds up on artery walls.

polyunsaturated fat: A healthier form of fat found in most vegetable oils.

psyllium: A high-fiber food derived from the husks of the seeds of the Plantago ovata. It absorbs water and can increase feelings of fullness.

pulmonary artery: The artery that carries oxygen-poor blood from the heart to the lungs to pick up blood.

radiofrequency ablation: Procedure in which radio frequency energy is used to scar the heart tissue responsible for abnormal impulses.

radionuclide ventriculography: A procedure that involves injecting radioactive material into the bloodstream to show how well the heart chambers work and how much blood is in the heart and to measure the ejection fraction; also known as multiple gated acquisition scan (MUGA).

refractory: Unresponsive to treatment.

right atrium: The part of the heart that collects oxygen-poor blood from two large veins and contracts to push it into the right ventricle.

right-sided heart failure: In congestive heart failure, when the heart doesn't pump blood as it should and blood pools in areas below the heart, including the liver, legs, feet, ankles, gastrointestinal tract, and arms.

right ventricle: The part of the heart that contracts to push oxygen-poor blood out of the heart to the lungs.

saturated fat: Unhealthy form of fat found in animal products that can contributes to plaque build up.

sinus node: The heart's pacemaker that regulates contraction.

sinus rhythm: The normal rhythm of the heart.

sphygmomanometer: A device that measures your blood pressure in millimeters of mercury (mm Hg).

stent: A tiny metal scaffolding inserted into an artery to hold it open.

stress test: An EKG while you walk on a treadmill or ride a stationary bicycle.

systolic heart failure: When the left ventricle does not contract or pump blood properly.

systolic pressure: Measures blood pressure when the heart contracts to push blood out; it is the higher number when pressure is measured.

transducer: A device used in ultrasound that produces high-frequency sound.

transesophageal echocardiogram (TEE): Procedure in which a scope is inserted through the mouth and lowered down the esophagus to obtain images of the heart.

trans-fatty acids: Unsaturated fats that have been hydrogenated to make them more stable; they increase total cholesterol and LDL cholesterol levels.

transthoracic echocardiogram (TEE): A procedure in which an instrument is inserted through your mouth and lowered down the esophagus to obtain images.

treadmill test: An EKG performed while you exercise on a treadmill; also called a stress test.

triglycerides: Blood fats that appear shortly after eating; eventually they're converted into cholesterol.

ventricle: Lower chambers of the heart.

visceral fat: Abdominal fat.

Notes

www.ingramcontent.com/pod-product-compliance
Lightning Source LLC
Chambersburg PA
CBHW030815180526
45163CB00003B/1295